How to be a Great Nurse –
The Heart of Nursing

For the full range of M&K Publishing books please visit our website:
www.mkupdate.co.uk

How to be a Great Nurse – The Heart of Nursing

Carolyn Mackintosh-Franklin and Julie Santy-Tomlinson

How to be a great nurse – the heart of nursing
Carolyn Mackintosh-Franklin and Julie Santy-Tomlinson
ISBN: 978-1-910451-12-0

First published 2020

British Library Cataloguing in Publication Data
A catalogue record for this book is available from the British Library

Notice

Clinical practice and medical knowledge constantly evolve. Standard safety precautions must be followed, but, as knowledge is broadened by research, changes in practice, treatment and drug therapy may become necessary or appropriate. Readers must check the most current product information provided by the manufacturer of each drug to be administered and verify the dosages and correct administration, as well as contraindications. It is the responsibility of the practitioner, utilising the experience and knowledge of the patient, to determine dosages and the best treatment for each individual patient. Any brands mentioned in this book are as examples only and are not endorsed by the publisher. Neither the publisher nor the authors assume any liability for any injury and/or damage to persons or property arising from this publication.

To contact M&K Publishing write to:

M&K Update Ltd · The Old Bakery · St. John's Street

Keswick · Cumbria CA12 5AS

Tel: 01768 773030

publishing@mkupdate.co.uk

www.mkupdate.co.uk

Designed and typeset by Mary Blood
Printed in Scotland by Bell & Bain, Glasgow

Contents

Preface

How to be a Great Nurse considers the big issues that currently impact on nursing practice, from the perspective of those within the profession, and those in need of nursing care. Nursing is more than a series of skills or tasks. and this book supports readers to identify what is really at the heart of nursing practice, and how an understanding of key values, attributes and skills can help individual student nurses, and those already qualified, to develop and sustain great nursing care. All nurses want to be great nurses and to work with a great team. For patients and their families, being cared for by great nurses is the ultimate caring experience.

Focusing on compassion and caring, the core personal values great nurses need and how they can build, develop and sustain skilled, patient-centred and effective practice, this book provides insights that will enable readers to develop an in-depth understanding of these key issues. It will also enable them to think deeply about their own personal and professional values, skills and attitudes towards patients and care, and to act on the results of reflection and learning.

Each chapter focuses on a particular element in the complex jigsaw of factors that all contribute to great nursing. The chapters are illustrated by real-world case studies, self-assessment tools and exercises that enable the reader to reflect and revisit specific aspects as their career and education progresses. Ideas for further reading and self-development are also provided.

Chapter 1 identifies the meaning of great nursing from a variety of perspectives, giving readers an opportunity to reflect on the roles of head, heart and hands, which underpin the ideals of nursing care. Chapter 2 focuses on the core values of nursing practice, from a professional perspective, but with a key emphasis on personal integrity. Chapters 3 and 4 provide readers with an opportunity to learn and reflect on the skills and emotional intelligence needed to be both a great nurse and an effective nurse, with an emphasis on communication and the reader's own individual learning needs.

Career progression and the support of other nurses are discussed in Chapters 5 and 6. Readers can explore the concept of resilience and reflect on their own aptitudes to support their own practice and that of others. In Chapter 7 many of these ideas are drawn together to support the reader to identify what others expect great nursing to look like. Looking at nursing practice from the perspective of those receiving care is essential, as it enables readers to deepen their own learning and reflect on their own practice, whilst allowing them to explore the true heart of nursing.

Nursing, and the world in which nurses practise, are subject to constant change. The final chapter in the book therefore considers the future of nursing, the new horizons that are currently opening up and the new roles nurses may develop and lead, to ensure that great nursing care moves forward to meet the highly varied requirements of future practice scenarios.

How to be a Great Nurse focuses on fundamental issues that are relevant to all nurses, across all countries, fields and areas of practice. It is essential reading for student nurses, qualified nurses, supervisors, assessors, managers and nurse academics, who all want the nursing profession to invest in the highest-quality care, supporting all nurses to be great nurses, firmly rooted in the real heart of nursing practice.

Chapter 1

The meaning of great nursing

Introduction

Deciding to become a nurse means choosing to join a challenging profession that holds an important and unique position within society, with high public expectations. Great nurses see nursing as a privilege, and they place the patient's experience at the centre of everything they do. They set out to be great nurses and strive to achieve that goal. This chapter aims to help the reader understand what great nursing means and how nurses should conduct themselves in their professional role.

The nature of great nursing – head, heart and hand

Becoming a great nurse begins with understanding what nursing is and what its values are. To fully appreciate the broad and complex activity that is nursing, it is important to recognise the meaning of nursing and to be able to explain it to patients and families so that they know what to expect from nurses. The International Council of Nursing (ICN) (2002) defines both 'nursing' and 'a nurse' (see Box 1.1), highlighting the breadth of what nurses do for people with diverse healthcare needs, for all age groups and within all communities. This helps nursing practitioners to describe what they do: how care is given; what knowledge, skills and education are needed; and what makes nursing a profession; as well as the professional and personal values that guide everything nurses do.

Box 1.1 International Council of Nursing (ICN) definitions of nursing and a nurse (2002)

Definition of nursing (short version)

'Nursing encompasses autonomous and collaborative care of individuals of all ages, families, groups and communities, sick or well and in all settings. Nursing includes the promotion of health, prevention of illness, and the care of ill, disabled and dying people. Advocacy, promotion of a safe environment, research, participation in shaping health policy and in patient and health systems management, and education are also key nursing roles.'

> **Definition of a nurse**
>
> 'The nurse is a person who has completed a program of basic, generalized nursing education and is authorized by the appropriate regulatory authority to practice nursing in his/her country. Basic nursing education is a formally recognized program of study providing a broad and sound foundation in the behavioural, life, and nursing sciences for the general practice of nursing, for a leadership role, and for post-basic education for specialty or advanced nursing practice. The nurse is prepared and authorized (1) to engage in the general scope of nursing practice, including the promotion of health, prevention of illness, and care of physically ill, mentally ill, and disabled people of all ages and in all healthcare and other community settings; (2) to carry out healthcare teaching; (3) to participate fully as a member of the healthcare team; (4) to supervise and train nursing and healthcare auxiliaries; and (5) to be involved in research.'

To understand what nurses need to know, and how they need to behave, in order to be effective care-givers, it is useful to explore nursing from three angles : the head, the heart and the hand. This framework, first discussed by Galvin and Todres (2011), can help us define effective nursing practice.

The hand

Nursing is, first and foremost, a practical activity involving specific activities and interventions that aim to improve the health and/or wellbeing of those receiving care. The range of practical tasks nurses undertake varies in complexity, from helping a patient to drink or wash themselves, to taking observations or being part of a team following a cardiac arrest or caring for someone who is dying – activities that often involve intimate contact with individuals who are experiencing distress. Such intimacy involves a holistic 'body, mind and social approach'. To carry out practical tasks and develop a meaningful relationship with the patient, the nurse's hands are often in physical contact with the patient's body as they provide physical care: hence, 'nursing with the hand' (Galvin & Todres 2011). Even seemingly simple interventions, such as helping someone to walk to the bathroom, can have a positive impact on health and recovery, depending on the way the task is carried out by the nurse.

Being in a person's personal space and touching their clothing or body is a natural part of the nursing role, but may be a source of fear, anxiety or embarrassment for the patient. Touch itself can be a way to bring comfort to people in distressing situations, depending on cultural norms. Offering a hand to hold, touching someone briefly to indicate closeness or empathy, for example. These are actions that are often reserved for close family members, and it may not be acceptable to the patient to be touched by someone they do not know. Nurses need a highly developed sense of when and how to touch someone. The nurse's hands are central to such activities. They are the tools used to carry out care and, although they can be used to provide comfort, they can also place the patient at risk of, for example, infection. It is important, therefore, that knowledge of how to carry out physical tasks safely and effectively is incorporated into each nurse's education and professional development throughout their careers.

The heart

Nursing is much more than simply 'doing' practical things for people. The way in which actions are carried out is what sets nursing apart from tasks performed by those who are not members of the caring professions. Physical nursing actions cannot be conducted in isolation from the emotional elements of the process of caring for people. Practical nursing care needs to be carried out in ways that least distress patients and reap the most therapeutic benefits. Nurses therefore need to engage with the people in their care with regard for them as individuals, considering the need for a humanistic approach that involves acting with compassion and treating the patient with dignity. Galvin and Todres (2011) call this 'nursing with the heart', signifying an approach to the patient that incorporates emotional engagement with their needs and experiences. It is argued that nursing with the heart is the most important aspect of being a great nurse – that it is possible to learn the skills and knowledge needed to provide acceptable nursing care, but that being able to engage with those in need in a heartfelt way is a more difficult talent to develop (unless the nurse has the right characteristics in the first place).

Nursing with the heart must include an appreciation of the rights of individuals to be cared for by nurses who make every attempt to empathise – to understand and engage with the experience of the person receiving care. This involvement of emotion and understanding is sometimes referred to as the 'art' of nursing. It is something that requires talent and cannot always be taught, and it requires someone who possesses the right personality or disposition in the first place. Recruiting the right kind of person to the nursing profession is an important part of ensuring that nurses have the right attitude towards others.

The head

Nursing is often described as both an 'art' and a 'science'. Along with interventions, and the emotional aspects of care, being a nurse involves having a distinct body of knowledge that is sometimes separate from, and sometimes aligned with, that of medical or allied health professional colleagues. Increasingly, nursing actions are based on what is known as 'evidence' – knowledge generated through rigorous research. Evidence helps professionals identify the best ways to do things and ensure that the actions they take are of maximum benefit to the patient. The notion of evidence-based practice will be considered in more detail in Chapter 3

Nursing can be viewed as a science because there are physical, psychological and social sciences that enable nurses to carry out their role in a manner that can improve health and wellbeing. Having a knowledge of biological sciences (such as anatomy, physiology and pathology) gives nurses an understanding of health and disease. This enables them to assess individuals and to select and carry out interventions with the aim of improving health and wellbeing, facilitating recovery and rehabilitation, and educating and empowering people and their families to take control of their own health.

However, the biological sciences alone are not a sufficient basis for good nursing practice. Nurses also need an understanding of the impact of social sciences and applied sciences (such as public health) to gain a full appreciation of how human beings work and how they interact with the world around them. Basing practice on the best available evidence ensures that nurses have the knowledge required to provide the best possible care in a way that directly meets their patients' needs. Great nurses apply this scientific understanding to the decisions they make when they provide care for patients. See Box 1.2 for an example of the application of the 'head, heart, hand' framework.

Box 1.2 An example of how the 'head, heart and hand' approach can facilitate good nursing

In an earlier paper discussing 'openheartedness' and its application to nursing, Galvin and Todres (2009) give some examples of care situations where great nursing is needed. Here is one example:

'A man of 45 is laid on his back in a hospital bed on an open ward with seven other patients. It is the middle of the day and meals are about to be served. He is lying in his faeces and he is in pain. He cannot move and is aware of the stench of his faeces and the presence of other patients. He has been like this for 5 minutes, but he knows the nurse is on his way; he has gone to get a bowl, cloths, and water. He feels a degree of self-disgust, even self-loathing; an overpowering anxiety, a deep worry that everyone around is also extremely averse to this situation and is bearing this smell resentfully. He wants to be invisible, not noticed.'

Thinking about this situation can be distressing – we can imagine how we might feel if we were this man, or a member of his family. Sadly, nurses become socialised to this kind of situation; because it is an event they commonly have to deal with, they may not engage with the patient's emotional distress at the time – simply undertaking the practical task of fetching the bowl and water and cleaning up the patient.

If we consider this vignette from the 'head, heart and hand' perspective, we can see how important it is not to simply act with the 'hand'. Being able to understand, with the 'head', the likely detrimental impact of this situation on the patient (from a physical, psychological and social perspective) enables the great nurse to use this knowledge when making decisions about how to act in the best way to preserve dignity, as far as possible.

However, none of this will be effective unless nurses also engage the 'heart' and empathise with the patient. Then nurses can use their own emotional intelligence to engage with the patient's distress and allow this to feed into their actions and the way they interact with the patient. This can lead to the (apparently) simple action of explaining to the patient why this distressing event has happened, that it isn't unusual, and that it is no trouble to help him to clean up. If the nurse does this in a way that is carefully worded, uses appropriate verbal and non-verbal communication skills, and takes account of the need to maintain as much privacy and dignity for the patient as possible, the patient may be less distressed. This takes a great deal of skill and, perhaps, talent.

Learning activity 1.1 Telling a story about hand, heart and head

Telling stories can help us understand our experiences of nursing practice.

Think about nursing, some of the people you have looked after and some of the nurses and other colleagues you have worked with. Based on these experiences, think about one incident where you have used a combination of hand, heart and head to provide nursing care.

Write the story down and focus on where you used hand, heart and head, and highlight how these aspects of nursing all worked together in this experience.

Questions:

- Did each element balance the other out?
- Or did you need a bit more of one than the other?
- What could you have done to ensure that all three elements were working together to provide the best possible nursing experience?

Nursing values – the characteristics of a great nurse

Baillie and Black (2015) identify values as a set of beliefs that influence behaviour. Such values can change over time, which suggests that they can be learnt and developed over time; and learning and developing values is one of the goals of nursing education. There are inherent links between values and ethics, which Sellman (2011) refers to as 'virtues' – meaning a moral or intellectual disposition that leads a person to act in a 'right and just' way. In recognising the vulnerability of those receiving care, morals, values and virtues become essential characteristics of any nurse (let alone a great one) if effective care is to be given and the public are to be protected from uncaring nursing.

'Caring' is a term that is often used synonymously with nursing, although people do not have to be professional nurses in order to 'care' for someone. Theorists and researchers have attempted to define numerous elements of caring over several decades. These are often based on the notion of humanism, a philosophical approach that considers individuals as whole people, rather than reducing them to, for example, an illness or a problem. When applied to nursing, humanism recognises that the behaviours and needs of human beings are complex and influenced by many factors, including their own experiences and concept of themselves (Paterson & Zderad 1974). Great nurses, characteristically, accept and engage with those in their care in a way that recognises the uniqueness of each person and uses this understanding to direct their caring practice.

Caring is behaviour that demonstrates compassion and respect for individuals (Cipriano 2007) and is the foundation of the professional values applied to nursing, a concept that will be referred to throughout this book. These values are based on moral conduct: behaving in a way towards others that is ethical and acknowledges the value of human beings. Some of the terms that are synonymous with caring have become the values and behaviours expected of good nurses. These are outlined in Table 1.1 and will be explored in more detail in Chapter 2.

Table 1.1 Common terminology used to describe nursing values and behaviours synonymous with caring

Value/behaviour	Meaning
Kindness	Recognising the needs of others and acting to meet those needs – often without being specifically asked to do so
Compassion	Understanding what people go through, especially when they are suffering, and adapting our own attitudes and behaviour towards them accordingly
Empathy	Engaging with the experiences of others and sharing in their experiences by considering what it is like to be them in their situation
Respect	Showing consideration for the thoughts, feelings, wishes, rights and needs of others
Trust/trustworthiness	Not only being honest and truthful, but being someone who can be relied upon to do what is right when needed
Being non-judgmental	Accepting of the differences between self and others, displaying respect and meeting the needs of others, regardless of those differences
Holism	Taking into account, and engaging with, the experiences and needs of the whole person, not just their physical needs; often linked to humanism
Being person-centered	Focused on the needs of people and the things that matter to them, including their physical, psychological, social, cultural and spiritual needs: often concerned with avoiding a focus on the needs of the carer or the care organisation
Professionalism	Being educated, competent and skilled in a specific profession so that a professional service of some kind can be provided for others, based on the standards, rules and values of that profession

These characteristics of nurses can be difficult to achieve consistently. Nurses often work in circumstances that can be physically, psychologically and emotionally difficult and they need to develop ways of coping with these circumstances at the same time as making sure they continue to practise effectively. This will be considered in more detail in Chapter 5.

Learning activity 1.2 What does 'caring' mean to you?

Many nursing textbooks and websites attempt to define what caring is and why it is so important in nursing. Some examples can be found in the further reading section at the end of this chapter.

However, this book aims to help you to understand your own approach to caring, as well as guiding you in your thinking. It is therefore helpful to begin to form your own ideas about what the term 'caring' means to you, and how it influences the way you think and behave, in preparation for considering this in more detail in Chapter 2:

1. To begin with, and before you undertake any further reading, write a few sentences about what caring means to you right now. Try to think of it in terms of your own behaviour, attitudes and

ideas about its meaning. What makes you a 'caring' person, suitable for the nursing profession? If you find this difficult, think about how 'caring' relates to the 'head, heart and hand' framework discussed earlier.

2. Once you have written down your own thoughts about caring and thought about it from your own perspective, do some research on 'caring' specifically applied to nursing. You could access some of the books recommended in the further reading section, or any of the general nursing texts that often consider this topic as part of a general introduction to nursing. You could also undertake a simple internet search combining terms such as 'caring' or 'care' and 'nurse' or 'nursing'. This will give you a general overview of what is currently seen as the caring role of the nurse and some of wider thinking on the topic, as well as (potentially) some news stories.

3. Think about, and make some notes on, your own perceptions of 'caring' and 'nursing' – and how both of these relate to your experiences of caring in your life so far.

How the history of nursing drives its present and future

Having an overview of the history of nursing is important in being able to see how the profession has become what it is, and visualise how it might develop in the future. Great nurses have been present at all levels and stages of societies at all times, from prehistory to the present day, although their skills have developed and matured as increasing knowledge has added to the scope of nursing practice. In prehistoric times, those who were ill or injured were cared for by others in their family or social group; and there is now considerable evidence that prehistoric man carried out a range of medical activities, including setting broken bones and basic surgical techniques such as trepanation (the deliberate making of holes in the skull). Skeletal remains suggest some success in these endeavours, with clear evidence of bone healing and associated implications for successful care.

As historical records have become available, evidence has grown to support the development of systematic practice which we now recognise as nursing care. Within Christian society, the development of religious orders in monasteries and convents, whose missions focused on care of the sick and poor, is extensively documented. The Knights Templar were one of the most famous of these; when not fighting, they were a nursing order, caring for the sick as well as those injured in battle.

In other societies, a culture of caring for the sick and injured was also promoted as a religious obligation, running parallel to the developments in medical knowledge led by early anatomists. This resulted in much greater understanding of how the body worked and, hence, reasons for illness and the first identification of possible cures.

Long periods of conflict, and the development of permanent standing armies, also helped drive the development of early nursing practice. As soldiers were injured in battle or became ill because of infectious diseases or poor hygiene, poor diet and lack of clean water, the need to care for them became apparent. Initially, informal camp followers were frequently used in nursing roles. Later they were replaced by orderlies – soldiers specifically trained for this purpose.

Outside the military or religious sphere, most societies had the equivalent of a 'wise woman' or 'wise man' who could be called upon at times of illness or injury to provide support. Some of this 'wise' activity was focused on childbirth, as well as on providing remedies (usually herbal) which could be used to alleviate symptoms.

The more formal development of nursing started to take place in Britain in the nineteenth century, with the beginnings of organised healthcare in voluntary hospitals, workhouse infirmaries and asylums for the insane. Initially, care within these institutions was provided by a variety of people. In the voluntary hospitals, specific staff were recruited as orderlies or domestic servants. In workhouse infirmaries, care was provided by the more able inmates, with strict sexual segregation, whereby male inmates cared for male patients, and women inmates cared for women and children. Within the asylums, physical strength was considered an important asset and male attendants, or keepers, were frequently recruited because of their ability to 'apply restraint'. This ad hoc approach to recruitment meant that nurses were not necessarily considered to be 'good' people or even 'good' at their role.

In 1848, writing about the character of the nurse Mrs Gamp in his novel *Martin Chuzzlewit*, Charles Dickens stated:

> '...it is notorious that the present race of hospital nurses do not come up to the standards of the very ideal of nurses – women of patience, gentleness and self-devotion of the kind of the sisters of charity. Mrs Gamp may well be a caricature, but her likeness is very traceable.' *(Fraser's Magazine 1848, in Williams 1974).*

Nearly 100 years later, in 1940, male naval nurses were described by Forster (Boorer 1968) as:

> 'men who deserved nothing better … who were ordered to do it on account of their incapacity or bad record, like men ordered to clean out latrines.'

Over time, it became widely recognised that this rather haphazard way of providing care did not lead to the best outcomes; and there were several campaigns for reform of the care of the physically and mentally ill and injured. Elizabeth Fry was a leading social reformer who brought about significant changes to the way those in prison and the poor were treated. She argued for a more humane perspective, opening the first nurse training school in 1840 and pioneering the development of what is now known as district or community nursing.

This would provide inspiration for the better-known nursing reformer Florence Nightingale who, after her well-documented work with soldiers in the Crimean war (using nurses trained in Fry's school), opened a similar nurse training school at St Thomas's Hospital in London in 1860. This is widely credited as the first non-religiously affiliated professional nurse training school in the world.

From this date onwards, nursing became a formidable and respected profession, with the principles first espoused by Florence Nightingale promoted and developed wherever professional nursing was practised. In the USA, the American Nursing Association (ANA) was founded in 1896 and, in the UK, the Royal College of Nursing was founded in 1916. Following the First World War, official recognition of the professional status of nursing in the UK was granted with the

1919 registration act and the creation of the General Nursing Council in 1920 (now the Nursing and Midwifery Council). Similar developments occurred across the globe, with the International Council of Nurses being founded in 1899, the Canadian Nursing Association being founded in 1908 and the Australian Nursing Federation in 1924.

History clearly demonstrates the progress that nursing as a profession has made towards humanistic ideals of care for the sick and vulnerable. The 'hand, heart and head' approach is directly linked to the evolution of the profession, inspired by the ideals of early nursing pioneers such as Elizabeth Fry and Florence Nightingale. The essential skills of 'hand, heart and head' therefore not only have a direct link with nursing's past but also play a fundamental part in shaping the future of nursing.

Further reading –
the history and development of the nursing profession

If you are interested in the background and history of the development of the nursing profession you may find some of the following resources and books interesting:

Borsay, A. & Hunter, B. (2012). *Nursing and Midwifery in Britain Since 1700.* Basingstoke: Palgrave Macmillan.

Bostridge, M. (2009). *Florence Nightingale, the Woman and the Legend.* Houndmills: Penguin

Dingwall, R., Rafferty, A.C. & Webster, C. (1988). *An Introduction to the Social History of Nursing.* London: Routledge.

Opperman, A.D. (2015). *While it is Yet Day: A Biography of Elizabeth Fry.* Leominster: Orphans Publishing.

The Royal College of Nursing (2020). History of Nursing Forum: https://www.rcn.org.uk/get-involved/forums/history-of-nursing-forum (last accessed 6.1.2020).

The UK Association for the History of Nursing: http://ukahn.org/wp/ (last accessed 6.1.2020).

Wyatt, L. (2019). *A history of nursing.* Stroud: Amberley Publishing.

Perceptions of nursing

The way nurses behave, and the attitudes of the public towards them, are led by perceptions of what nurses do and how they do it. These perceptions have developed over many years and are an integral part of nursing's history and pedigree. Images of nurses and nursing, both past and present, are an important part of how patients and families perceive nurses and the care they provide as well as their confidence in accessing nursing services. The public image of nursing is also important because it has an impact on recruitment to the profession as well as on nurses' satisfaction in their work (Takase *et al.* 2006).

Although, in the past (especially before the nineteenth century), nurses have not always been perceived as 'good' humans (as discussed above), the public perception of them has been consistently positive over the last century or more. However, there are several aspects of the public image of nursing that demonstrate the fragility of these perceptions, as seen in public and media responses to failures in care in which nurses have been implicated (see Box 1.4 for some examples of cases in which care failures, abuse and neglect have been highlighted).

It is upsetting to have to consider these cases of very poor standards of nursing practice in a book about great nursing, but it is also important for nurses and the nursing profession to learn from the mistakes that have been made. When the media focuses on failures in healthcare (see Box 1.4) there is often an emphasis on concerns about standards of nursing. Girvin *et al.* (2016) explored this issue and found that the media have recently portrayed nursing, particularly in the UK, as a troubled profession and have tended to demean the profession. This review suggested that although nursing was a trusted profession, it was not respected by the public in the same way as, for example, the medical profession. It has been suggested that part of the problem is that the roles and benefits of nursing are poorly understood. The public do not, for example, understand how nursing education works, nor are they aware of the 'unseen' work nurses do when preparing to give care, developing skills and expertise and maintaining their knowledge and competence.

The reasons that individuals choose a career in nursing vary, and there is often an element of wanting to help others, although these decisions are sometimes made for more complex reasons. Perceptions of the role of the nurses, from both a clinical activity perspective and an emotional perspective, are often led by previous experiences of being involved in caring or seeing caring taking place. Historical, media and societal portrayals of nursing, particularly on television and social media, can also have an impact. However, the reality of the day-to-day role of the nurse can be quite different from prior perceptions and this can result in disappointment and, sometimes, leaving the profession.

Partly due to the early religious origins of nursing, society generally expects nurses to be more interested in fulfilling their role than the financial reward they receive. Payment has therefore often been portrayed as a secondary reason for entering the nursing profession. However, this attitude is unrealistic in modern society.

Box 1.4 Examples of well-publicised failures in nursing

The following examples illustrate the vulnerability of people receiving nursing care and how nurses can be instrumental in upholding standards of healthcare.

Mid Staffordshire Foundation NHS Trust
An inquiry (Francis 2013) into poor standards and failures in care that occurred in one UK NHS Trust between 2005 and 2008 found that there were several areas where compassionate, safe nursing culture (as well as other aspects of care) was not always upheld and that patients and their families suffered as a result. Poor practice had become accepted and basic nursing care had been neglected. This report and its implications have had far-reaching effects on the public's perception of healthcare and nurses. Many changes have been put in place since that time, but shocking failures in care have continued to be highlighted across the UK and beyond.

Winterbourne View Hospital
In 2012 the UK Department of Health published a report into abuse, by nurses and other healthcare workers, of vulnerable children, young people and adults with learning disabilities, autism and mental health problems. Staff failed in their duty of care and criminally mistreated, abused and neglected those whom they should have been protecting from harm. A programme of action is needed to transform services for people with learning difficulties.

Gosport War Memorial Hospital
Over many years, families' concerns about the care of their loved ones receiving palliative and end-of-life care at the War Memorial Hospital were ignored. The report of the Gosport War Memorial Independent Panel (2018) highlighted failings in the way in which nurses' concerns were ignored regarding the prescribing and administration of dangerous doses of drugs to patients for whom they were not clinically justified. These drugs caused the unnecessary death of patients. When nurses attempted to raise their concerns about medical practice, they were ignored and/or action was not taken by the appropriate authorities.

Even though nurses have been involved in these events, and the nursing profession has itself questioned whether the 'care' aspects of nursing are being lost (McSherry, McSherry & Watson 2012), the confidence of the public in nurses and what they do remains high and nurses are often presented in the media as the most trusted of professionals. Nevertheless, there have also been high-profile cases of nurses who have sought to deliberately harm others while carrying out their professional duties. The need to protect the public from lack of professionalism, and from those who could misuse the privileged position of nurses working with those who are vulnerable, is enshrined in law and regulation in most countries.

Learning activity 1.3 The public image of nursing

- Undertake a search of the Internet for positive and negative stories or portrayals of nursing or nurses.
- Select one positive portrayal of nursing or nurses and one negative portrayal to reflect on and consider in more detail.
- Was it easier to find negative portrayals or positive ones? Why do you think that might be?
- Would you say that the media portrayals of nursing are full and accurate representations of what nurses do?
- What are your own feelings about this?
- What do you think the nursing profession needs to do to make sure the public perception of nurses and nursing is as accurate as possible?

Professionalism, professional identity and public protection

Nursing has been referred to as a profession since the mid-twentieth century. Professionals are people who carry out respected roles within society, such as members of the legal and medical/health professions and teachers. There are several characteristics that all these professions have in common, including public service, professional autonomy, a scientific basis for practice, university-level education, bespoke skills, and a commitment to competence and continuous education.

Professional regulation is another marker for professionalism. In the UK, such regulation is currently overseen by the Nursing and Midwifery Council (NMC) whose role has developed to include protection of the public by making sure nurses (as well as midwives and associate nurses) have the skills they need to care for people effectively. The NMC is a regulating body that can take action if concerns are raised about the standards of a nurse's practice. *The Code*, published by the NMC (2015), is a guide to professional conduct that lays out for nurses, and for the public they serve, the minimum standards of professional behaviour and practice that can be expected of every nurse – its main elements are outlined in Table 1.2.

In the UK, the NMC governs registration of all nurses and the education standards they must meet to be registered practitioners. If a nurse fails to meet the expected standards of conduct and professionalism, the NMC's conduct committee can choose to suspend or remove them from the register so that they can no longer practise as a registered nurse. *The Code* needs to be studied in detail as it describes each of the standards in depth, is easily accessed online and should be part of the everyday life of a nurse. It includes some aspects that are not only integral to the behaviour of a nurse when carrying out their professional duties, but also in their day-to-day lives. *The Code* is also a fundamental part of nursing education programmes, and student nurses and learner associate nurses are expected to incorporate it into all elements of what they do.

Table 1.2 The elements of the professional standards within the NMC Code (2015)

NMC professional standard	Elements of the standard
Prioritise people	1. Treat people as individuals and uphold their dignity 2. Listen to people and respond to their preferences and concerns 3. Make sure that people's physical, social and psychological needs are assessed and responded to 4. Act in the best interests of people at all times 5. Respect people's right to privacy and confidentiality
Practise effectively	6. Always practise in line with the best available evidence 7. Communicate clearly 8. Work co-operatively 9. Share your skills, knowledge and experience for the benefit of people receiving care and your colleagues 10. Keep clear and accurate records relevant to your practice 11. Be accountable for your decisions to delegate tasks and duties to other people 12. Have in place an indemnity arrangement which provides appropriate cover for any practice you take on as a nurse, midwife or nursing associate in the United Kingdom
Preserve safety	13. Recognise and work within the limits of your competence 14. Be open and candid with all service users about aspects of care and treatment, including when any mistakes or harm have taken place

cont.	15. Always offer help if an emergency arises in your practice setting or anywhere else
	16. Act without delay if you believe there is a risk to patient safety or public protection
	17. Raise concerns immediately if you believe a person is vulnerable or at risk and needs extra support and protection
	18. Advise on, prescribe, supply, dispense or administer medicines within the limits of your training and competence, the law, our guidance and other relevant policies, guidance and regulations
	19. Be aware of, and reduce as far as possible, any potential for harm associated with your practice
Promote professionalism and trust	20. Uphold the reputation of your profession at all times
	21. Uphold your position as a registered nurse, midwife or nursing associate
	22. Fulfil all registration requirements
	23. Cooperate with all investigations and audits
	24. Respond to any complaints made against you professionally
	25. Provide leadership to make sure people's wellbeing is protected and to improve their experience of the health and care system

This model of regulation, comprising the use of professional registers and codes of conduct, has been followed globally, with all countries in the developed world and most countries in the developing world hosting their own professional regulatory body and bespoke standards of practice. Further information about other countries' professional regulation is held by the International Council of Nurses in their role as the worldwide representative of the nursing profession (see ICN list of regulatory bodies https://www.icn.ch/sites/default/files/inline-files/ Regulatory%20bodies_database-1-7.pdf).

It's important to recognise that nurses rarely work in isolation; rather they work with other members of health and social care teams who collaboratively assess the patient, and plan, implement and evaluate care based on patient needs and the collective skills of the team. These teams are often referred to as multidisciplinary or interdisciplinary teams to reflect the collaboration and mutual respect needed for them to operate effectively in the best interests of the individuals and communities they work with. It has been consistently demonstrated that effective multidisciplinary team working has a positive impact on patient outcomes, especially in relation to aspects of healthcare where patient needs are complex. Some aspects of multidisciplinary team working are considered in Chapter 4.

Conclusion

An understanding of what nursing is, and how it has developed, is key to being able to articulate the value of what nurses do and how they do it. Great nurses practise their craft with the patient at the centre of what they do, embodying a humanistic approach. To be successful, nurses need a set of professional values that contribute to caring in a way that acknowledges the value of nursing with the hand, the head and the heart. Learning to care in a way that incorporates all of these is central to become a great professional nurse. However, the public image of nursing and nurses in the UK has been affected by some well-publicised 'failures in care'. This underlines the importance of nurses being regulated by their professional body and has enabled the ongoing focus on caring values and professional behaviour of all great nurses.

The key points from this chapter can best be summarised in six principles for all great nurses (see Box 1.5).

Box 1.5 How to be a great nurse – six principles

1. Examine your own motivation for being a nurse, bearing in mind what nursing is and what it means to those receiving nursing care.

2. Develop and seek to continuously develop the practical tasks of nursing – nursing with the 'hand'.

3. Nurse with the 'heart' – engage emotionally with those for whom you provide care so that you develop a positive therapeutic relationship with them.

4. Work towards career-long learning, so that the knowledge you need to nurse with the 'head' is constantly kept up to date and used in your practice

5. Study the professional *Code* (NMC 2015) so that you are fully aware of what is expected of you.

6. Ask yourself if you have the capacity to be a great nurse and think about what you need to do to make it happen.

Recommendations for further study

Baillie, L. & Black S. (2015). *Professional values in nursing.* London: CRC Press.

Baughan, J. & Smith, A. (2013). *Compassion, caring and communication: Skills for nursing practice.* 2nd edn. Harlow: Pearson.

Galvin, K. & Todres, L. (2012). *Caring and well-being: A lifeworld approach.* London: Routledge.

References

Baillie, L. & Black S. (2015). *Professional values in nursing.* London: CRC Press.

Boorer D, J. (1968) Man nurses in Britain. *Nursing Outlook.* 16.11.24-26

Department of Health (2012). *Transforming care: A national response to Winterbourne View Hospital.* https://assets.publishing.service.gov.uk/government/uploads/system/uploads/attachment_data/file/213215/final-report.pdf (last accessed 7.1.2020).

Cipriano, P. (2007). Celebrating the art and science of nursing. *American Nurse Today.* **2**(5), 8.

Francis, R. (2013). *Report of the Mid Staffordshire NHS Foundation Trust Public Enquiry. Executive summary.* https://webarchive.nationalarchives.gov.uk/20150407084231/http://www.midstaffspublicinquiry.com/report (last accessed 7.1.2020).

Galvin, K.T. & Todres, L. (2009). Embodying nursing openheartedness: An existential perspective. *Journal of Holistic Nursing.* **27**(2), 141–49.

Galvin, K.T. & Todres, L. (2010). Research based empathic knowledge for nursing: A translational strategy for disseminating phenomenological research findings to provide evidence for caring practice. *International Journal of Nursing Studies.* Published Online. DOI:10.1016/j.ijnurstu.2010.08.009.

Girvin, J., Jackson, D. & Hutchison, M. (2016). Contemporary public perceptions of nursing: a systematic review and narrative synthesis of the international research evidence. *Journal of Nursing Management.* **24**(8) 994–1006. https://doi.org/10.1111/jonm.12413

Gosport Independent Panel (2018). *Gosport War Memorial Hospital: The report of the Gosport Independent Panel.* https://www.gosportpanel.independent.gov.uk/media/documents/070618_CCS207_CCS03183220761_Gosport_Inquiry_Whole_Document.pdf (last accessed 7.1.2020).

International Council of Nurses (ICN) (2002). *Definition of Nursing.* https://www.icn.ch/nursing-policy/nursing-definitions (last accessed 7.1.2020).

McSherry, W., McSherry, R. & Watson, R. (2012). *Care in nursing. Principles, values and skills.* Oxford: Oxford University Press.

Nursing and Midwifery Council (NMC) (2015). *The Code: Professional standards of practice and behaviour for nurses, midwives and nursing associates.* https://www.nmc.org.uk/globalassets/sitedocuments/nmc-publications/nmc-code.pdf (last accessed 7.1.2020).

Paterson, J. & Zderad, L. (1976). *Humanistic nursing.* New York: John Wiley.

Sellman, D. (2011). *What makes a good nurse: Why the virtues are important for nurses.* London: Jessica Kingsley.

Takase, M., Maude, P. & Manias, E. (2006). Impact of the perceived public image of nursing on nurses' work. *Journal of Advanced Nursing.* **53**(3), 333–43.

Williams, K. (1974). 'Ideologies of nursing: their meanings and implications' in: *Readings in the Sociology of Nursing.* Edinburgh: Churchill Livingstone.

Chapter 2

Core values for nursing

Introduction

The evolution of the nursing profession, with its central focus on the principles of 'hand, heart and head' (discussed in Chapter 1), has had a continuous impact on the development of nursing and the current core values which are central to best practice in the twenty-first century. However, given the range of recent failings in care (see Chapter 1, Box 1.4), how well these essential characteristics have been embedded in nursing practice remains open to question. These failings have forced the profession to look seriously at its own practice and how well current core values are reflected in the actual activities of registered nurses.

It is important to note that these core values are not static, and current values have developed to keep pace with several contemporary issues: the times, the general needs of the profession, its place within the overall context of healthcare, and the needs, expectations and perceptions of people receiving nursing care. Current perceptions have moved a long way from the early ad hoc, and religious origins of nursing and closer to the secular humanistic values which form the characteristics of professional caring disciplines today.

Current core values

The current core values of the nursing profession can be articulated in several largely context-specific ways. In the United States (US), the National League for Nurses (NLN) identifies four core values:

1. **Caring:** promoting health, healing and hope in response to the human condition
2. **Integrity:** respecting the dignity and moral wholeness of every person without conditions or limitation
3. **Diversity:** affirming the uniqueness of, and differences among, persons, ideas, values and ethnicities
4. **Excellence:** co-creating and implementing transformative strategies with daring ingenuity.

In the United Kingdom (UK), the Royal College of Nursing (RCN 2018) has promoted the use of eight core principles underpinning best practice (see Box 2.1).

Box 2.1 Royal College of Nursing eight core principles underpinning best practice

Principle A: Nurses and nursing staff treat everyone in their care with dignity and humanity – they understand their individual needs, show compassion and sensitivity and provide care in a way that respects all people equally.

Principle B: Nurses and nursing staff take responsibility for the care they provide and answer for their own judgements and actions – they carry out these actions in a way that is agreed with their patients, and the families and carers of their patients, and in a way that meets the requirements of their professional bodies and the law.

Principle C: Nurses and nursing staff manage risk, are vigilant about risk, and help to keep everyone safe in the places they receive healthcare.

Principle D: Nurses and nursing staff provide and promote care that puts people at the centre, involves patients, service users, their families and their carers in decisions and helps them make informed choices about their treatment and care.

Principle E: Nurses and nursing staff are at the heart of the communication process: they assess, record and report on treatment and care, handle information sensitively and confidentially, deal with complaints effectively, and are conscientious in reporting the things they are concerned about.

Principle F: Nurses and nursing staff have up-to-date knowledge and skills, and use these with intelligence, insight and understanding in line with the needs of each individual in their care.

Principle G: Nurses and nursing staff work closely with their own team and with other professionals, making sure patients' care and treatment is co-ordinated, is of a high standard and has the best possible outcome.

Principle H: Nurses and nursing staff lead by example, develop themselves and other staff, and influence the way care is given in a manner that is open and responds to individual needs.

Alongside these principles, the National Health Service (NHS) in England (2018) promotes six key nursing values, known as the 'Six Cs':

1. Care
2. Compassion
3. Competence
4. Communication
5. Courage
6. Commitment.

Although these values use different terminology, the underpinning themes are consistent, emphasising the following attributes:

● Care and the actions of caring in a compassionate way
● Respect for the dignity of those receiving nursing care

- Non-judgemental understanding of diverse individuals and their different needs
- High levels of competence in the delivery and development of care
- Personal integrity and professional conduct
- Valuing the self.

These core values are at the heart of nursing and are central to the provision of excellence in nursing care and practice. Without them, nursing care will fall short, the experience of those using nursing services will suffer, and both the profession and individuals within the nursing profession will be compromised.

Learning activity 2.1 Telling a story of nursing values

Telling stories can be useful in helping us understand our experiences of caring (Baillie & Black 2015).

Looking at the values identified above by the NLN, the RCN and the NHS, choose one of the values/behaviours that you can illustrate with a story from your own experience. This could be an experience where you have received kindness or compassion, for example, or it could be an example of a time when you have demonstrated empathy or non-judgemental behaviour towards someone else.

Write the story down in detail, highlighting the little things that happened, or what someone said or did, that illustrate the value you have chosen.

At the end of the story, try to write a short conclusion about the meaning of the value/s or behaviour/s on which the story is based.

Care and the actions of caring compassionately

The two elements – care and compassion – are generally considered as interrelated parts of the same set of professional values. In a similar way to the concepts of Hand, Heart and Head introduced in Chapter 1, the word 'care' has a dual meaning in nursing practice:

1. To care in the physical sense – carrying out activities that demonstrate functional care (HAND)

2. To care in an emotional sense – showing empathetic or compassionate feelings for people needing nursing interventions (HEART).

Compassion is best defined as being sensitive to the needs of others, in a sympathetic and empathetic manner (HEART).

This dual meaning of care can be problematic, as the two elements are sometimes confused, and it can be difficult to define the actual qualities recognised as high-quality nursing 'care'. However, it is clear from the history of nursing and its current core values that 'care' is a long-established and fundamental element of best practice. It is also well-recognised that an absence of care in one or both forms leads to a reduction in standards of nursing practice and negative patient experiences (see Chapter 1, Box 1.4). The dual nature of 'care', and the common inability to clearly articulate how it can be identified and practised, can result in misunderstanding and unrealistic expectations on the part of nurses and other healthcare professionals as well as those in need of nursing 'care', and can have a major impact on public perceptions of nursing, as identified in Chapter 1.

In order to be great and caring nurses, it is essential that nurses themselves can identify exactly what care and compassion in nursing practice are, and how these qualities can be manifested in what they do.

Many different types of caring have been identified as relevant to nursing (Mackintosh 2000). Care is clearly not confined to nursing but is a fundamental emotional human attribute that we are all capable of demonstrating. Furthermore, care is closely linked to a moral or ethical dimension, which makes it possible for someone working in nursing to be considered virtuous by the simple nature of their work.

Recently, there has been some focus on the concept of emotional intelligence. This is best defined as the way in which an individual is able to process emotions (both their own and those experienced by others), and to act accordingly. In other words, emotional intelligence refers to the way in which someone is able to respond to and interpret their own and other people's emotional responses in any given situation. There is a growing body of evidence suggesting that people with higher levels of emotional intelligence are able to perform better in a wide range of situations because their work performance is enhanced. They also have better leadership skills and higher levels of job satisfaction, as well as a greater personal ability to cope with stress and avoid burnout (for further reading, you could look at Smith *et al.* 2009, Winship 2010, Adams & Iseler 2014).

It is also becoming increasingly evident that people with higher levels of emotional intelligence are more naturally inclined to provide more appropriate, responsive, compassionate care and to be great nurses. Nurses with higher levels of emotional intelligence may simply be better at responding to patients' needs and expressing empathetic caring behaviours as needed. This translates into better use of the 'heart', improved clinical practice performance and greater overall satisfaction amongst patients with the care they receive (Beauvais *et al.* 2011, Rankin 2013).

Functional care (HAND) is best recognised in the actions nurses perform each day: helping a patient meet their fundamental activities of daily living, carrying out a specific task such as a wound dressing, or taking on an advisory role such as assessment, health promotion or screening. Providing effective and efficient functional care cannot be divorced from providing compassionate, empathetic care (HEART), as the two go hand in hand. This means that the way in which a nurse undertakes a task has a major influence on outcomes, experiences and perceptions of care; and the emotionally intelligent nurse will readily recognise the benefits of responding appropriately and compassionately to each individual situation.

A useful way of thinking about care and compassion is to consider them as part of a relationship between those providing care and those needing it. This fits well with the person-centred approach to nursing, which assumes that the relationship between nurse and patient is two-way, or reciprocal. However, most nurses recognise that this is not always the case in practice. Not all people seek, want or are grateful for nursing care, and in some areas of nursing practice it is simply not possible to form a meaningful reciprocal relationship, due to a shortage of time and other environmental constraining factors (see Chapter 4 for further discussion about communication and the nurse-patient relationship). Emotionally intelligent responses can offer a good basis for navigating these difficulties and developing the appropriate relationship for each individual and situation.

One of the most straightforward methods of achieving high standards of care is to listen to what those needing care think and feel, and what they expect to receive. The failure of nursing and nurses to take account of care users' expectations frequently leads to misunderstandings and even breakdowns in the nurse-patient relationship. Studies that have focused on the care needs of patients, compared to the way nurses perceive those care needs, have consistently identified a divergence between the two. Patients' expectations tend to focus on care illustrated by clinical expertise and competence, linked to straightforward and honest open communication (HAND), while nurses often focus on demonstrating care by building relationships and providing empathetic emotional support (HEART) (Larsson *et al.* 1998). Patient perceptions of great nursing care are considered in detail in Chapter 7.

Learning activity 2.2 Using Hand and Heart to meet expectations of care and compassion

Telling stories can be useful in helping us understand our experiences of caring (Baillie & Black 2015), because patients' expectations of care are sometimes different from the expectations of the nurses providing the care.

- Think about some of the patients you may have met and the care you provided for them.
- Write down something about what you think those patients may actually have expected.
- How realistic do you think those expectations were? And how closely did they match your own?
- Think back to one key patient or experience; how did you meet that patient's expectations of care?

Respect for the dignity of those receiving nursing care

Dignity is an internationally recognised human right, enshrined within the Universal Declaration of Human Rights which was signed by 50 member countries of the United Nations in 1948. It is legally protected in the United Kingdom and Europe by the 1998 Human Rights Act (for more information see: https://www.equalityhumanrights.com/en/human-rights/what-are-human-rights). Respect for an individual's dignity is a key aspect of quality of life, not just for nursing and healthcare practice.

Within nursing, the preservation of dignity is a core component of practice, as nurses work closely with people who are frequently highly vulnerable and exposed to a range of procedures and experiences which can be greatly detrimental to maintaining personal dignity. People are also expected to communicate potentially intimate details about their lifestyle and health needs to professionals who are usually complete strangers, within an unfamiliar environment. Maintaining personal dignity in such situations can be difficult and all nurses need to recognise their own role in supporting individuals' right to dignity in all circumstances.

Consequently, dignity is a core value which is integral to high-quality nursing practice and it is enshrined in the American Nurses Association (ANA) code of ethics. It means to: 'treat people as individuals and uphold their dignity' and is the first standard in the NMC code of professional conduct (2015) (see Chapter 1). Its origins can be found in the Latin word *dignus* which contains the two related concepts of worth and respect and is generally understood as behaving towards people as if they are someone who is 'worthy of honour or respect' (Clark 2010). This definition has led the American Association of Colleges of Nursing (AACN) (2008) to define human dignity as 'the respect for the inherent worth and uniqueness of individuals and populations'.

Dignity is clearly a far-ranging concept that includes the principles of respect, autonomy, holism and empowerment, and encompasses the need for clear and accurate communication. However, as with the concept of care, dignity can be a difficult concept to grasp, due to its multidimensionality. An individual may possess dignity and yet people can be stripped of their dignity and have their dignity violated. This means that dignity is something that people experience by being treated in a dignified manner, which leads directly to individual differences in expectations regarding dignity, both in receiving and delivering dignified nursing care.

A useful way to move forward with this conundrum was suggested by Clark (2010) who considers dignity as having two aspects: the objective and the subjective. The objective aspect relates to the concept of human rights, and the central place of dignity as a core aspect of every individual's human experience. However, subjective dignity focuses on the individual and how they experience dignity, so this can be extended to consider an individual's own self-regard – in other words, how they feel about themselves and how they are perceived by others. The subjective experience of dignity has significant implications for nursing practice, as there can sometimes be a misalignment between an individual's expectations of dignified care (based on their own sense of worth and personal values) and those of the individual nurse.

This misalignment in expectations led Allen and Dennis (2009) to launch a Dignity in Care Campaign after witnessing these problems first-hand and reading the personal reports published by the Patients Association (PA 2020) which provide numerous examples of poor nursing practice violating the individual's right to meaningful, dignified care. These include instances where patients were denied basic human needs, such as timely and effective assistance with toileting and feeding, as well as being treated in degrading and disrespectful ways.

Allen and Dennis (2009) conclude their discussion by summarising key points about what constitutes best practice when providing dignified nursing care. These include:

- Dignity as a standard by which people measure their own conduct and that of others
- Recognition that those who do not provide dignified care, lack dignity themselves
- Emphasis on the statutory and moral duty of all healthcare workers to provide dignified care and protect people from any form of abuse.

The Dignity in Care Campaign suggests 10 Dignity Do's (see Box 2.2).

Box 2.2 Dignity in Care Campaign – 10 Dignity Do's

1. Have zero tolerance for all forms of abuse
2. Support people with the same respect you would want for yourself or a member of your family
3. Treat each person as an individual by offering a personalised service
4. Enable people to maintain the maximum possible level of independence, choice and control
5. Listen and support people to express their needs and wants
6. Respect people's rights to dignity
7. Ensure people feel able to complain without fear of retribution
8. Engage with family members and carers as care partners
9. Assist people to maintain confidence and positive self-esteem
10. Act to alleviate people's loneliness and isolation

(Taken from: Allen & Dennis 2009)
https://www.dignityincare.org.uk/About/The_10_Point_Dignity_Challenge/

These Dignity Do's link well with the Royal College of Nursing guidance (RCN 2016) on preserving dignity, which stresses that the behaviour of the individual nurse is always the biggest factor in maintaining someone's dignity, in any situation. The nurse's personal attitude, the manner in which they approach and speak to a person, and the level at which they engage with that individual, are all essential in practising dignified nursing care (in both its objective and subjective sense). These aspects could be deemed trivial, and are sometimes too easily forgotten, in the rush of a busy healthcare environment, but they are essential to providing a positive experience for both patients and nurses, and maintaining human dignity as central to great nursing care.

Learning activity 2.3 Maintaining dignity

Think about a recent experience of physical care which could be considered undignified – for example, providing personal care, or toileting help.

- Think of four ways in which you tried to maintain the patient's dignity whilst you were doing this and write them down.
- Now think about what else you could have done and try to list a further four ways in which you could have improved the experience for that patient. Remember, these can use both Hand and Heart.

Non-judgemental understanding of diverse individuals' different needs

The International Council of Nurses (ICN) (2012) Code of Ethics highlights the need for nursing care to be 'respectful of and unrestricted by considerations of age, colour, creed, culture, disability or illness, gender, sexual orientation, nationality, politics, race or social status' (ICN 2012, p. 1), and there is a tacit understanding that a core value of the nursing profession is the ability of nurses to work in a non-judgemental and non-discriminatory way.

However, being truly non-judgemental is not easy and one of the purposes of the professional education of qualified nurses is to raise and deepen their understanding of the need to both recognise and set aside their personal judgements and prejudices and fully adopt a professional non-judgemental approach. This does not mean that nurses should be blinded to individual differences; it simply means that nurses should have a clear understanding of their own views and attitudes towards others, so that these attitudes can be recognised and, where necessary, set aside.

Non-judgemental understanding applies to all aspects of nurses' work, including their relationships with all members of the workplace team, their direct and indirect clinical environment, and relationships with every individual, regardless of status. The expectation of non-judgemental respect should also extend beyond the workplace; for example, incidents where nurses have posted culturally disparaging posts on social media sites have led to professional disciplinary action and have sometimes resulted in nurses being removed from their professional register (see NMC disciplinary hearings: https://www.nmc.org.uk/concerns-nurses-midwives/hearings/hearings-sanctions/).

There is also an expectation that nurses will not only be non-judgemental, but will also be pro-active in taking positive action to remedy judgemental or prejudicial behaviour when they witness it (NMC 2010):

> 'All nurses must practise in a holistic, non-judgemental, caring and sensitive manner that avoids assumptions, supports social inclusion; recognises and respects individual choice; and acknowledges diversity. Where necessary, they must challenge inequality, discrimination and exclusion from access to care.'

When considering non-judgemental behaviour and attitudes within the nursing profession, it becomes clear that the background of qualified nurses is continuously changing. Evidence from the United States suggests that the nursing workforce is more culturally and ethnically diverse than ever before, with greater numbers of ethnic minority groups attaining baccalaureate graduate status and increased numbers of male entrants to the profession (Kovner *et al.* 2018, Zangaro *et al.* 2018). Although there is no directly observable correlation, the trend towards more diversity in the nursing profession is mirrored by changes in wider society. Within the UK, around 87 % of the population are classed as white, with the remaining 13 % coming from Black, Asian or mixed-race groups, with considerable regional variation in London (the capital), where 40.2 % of the population are from Black, Asian or mixed-race groups (Ethnicity facts and figures 2018). In the USA, however, around 72 % of the population were classed as white in the most recent 2010 census and the remainder, Black, Asian, Hispanic or mixed-race groups (Census 2010).

This means nurses have a duty to take a culturally competent, non-judgemental approach towards both their colleagues and those in receipt of nursing care. This will, almost certainly, present a challenge for many people, not necessarily as a result of prejudice. Sometimes the real challenge is for nursing education and training to provide culturally relevant knowledge, information and resources, so that nurses come to regard people as individuals from a particular culture, rather than as a generic representation of their cultural group.

Cultural diversity is by no means the only way in which individuals may differ from each other, although it is the most common reason for nurses to hold prejudicial or judgemental attitudes. Other sources of prejudice include, for example:

- Generational prejudice against older patients and older colleagues (also known as ageism)
- Prejudice against others on the basis of gender identity
- Prejudice against those with mental health conditions, learning or cognitive difficulties
- Prejudice against those who are overweight or obese
- Prejudice against those who contribute to their own ill-health through lifestyle choices, e.g. smokers and illicit drug users.

Despite all these possible differences, nurses need to be non-judgemental in their personal and professional lives at all times. Enhanced education, the adoption of non-judgemental professional work values and raising individuals' awareness of their own potential prejudices, can all make a positive difference when attempting to overcome judgemental views.

Great nurses will always be faced with challenging situations. For instance, they will encounter people who continue to undertake high-risk activities such as smoking, drinking or drug use despite medical advice. They will also have patients and colleagues who over-eat to the point of health-threatening obesity, and those whose social or cultural upbringing has given them differing and sometimes challenging sets of values, behaviours or norms which may be very different from their own. These challenges are not insurmountable but individual nurses must be sensitive to and aware of their own views and attitudes so that, when required, these can be put to one side. This will allow great nurses to take a non-judgemental stance towards the people they work with, and those diverse individuals who are in need of the highest standards of nursing care.

High levels of competence in the delivery and development of care

Being competent is generally considered to be a prerequisite for great nursing care. Surprisingly, however, there is no single accepted definition of a competent nurse. There is a general assumption that for someone to be competent, they must be capable of performing the skills needed to undertake their role (both HAND and HEAD). However, these skills can be highly variable between professions. Being a competent nurse may encompass a broad range of attributes, including performance in a set task, communication skills, leadership skills and overall attitude. Within nursing practice, there are two main aspects to competence. The first is a focus on specific skills or tasks, such as the ability to undertake a skill such as giving an intramuscular injection in a competent manner (the Hand). The second, more holistic, approach is where someone's competence is based on a wider cluster of activities, which can include more abstract concepts such as decision-making and critical thinking (Hand, Heart and Head together) (National Nursing Research Unit 2009).

In the UK, the NMC regularly publishes updated standards of competence for both qualified nurses and student nurses, which are the guiding principles by which competence in role performance can be judged (NMC 2019). For student nurses, these competencies can form the basis on which academic and clinical assessment performance can be gauged. Meanwhile, for qualified staff, they can be used as a benchmark to inform individual performance targets or as a basis for developing policy or clinical protocols. The NMC standards for registered nurses (2019) offer a fusion of the Hand, Head and Heart, from task-specific standards to a more holistic approach to competency, by focusing on four main areas of nursing practice applicable to all areas of nursing work:

- Professional values
- Communication and interpersonal skills
- Nursing practice and decision making
- Leadership, management and team working.

A key element in reaching and maintaining competence is the individual nurse's personal responsibility to be conscious of their own practice abilities and to recognise the demands of their role and profession and their own individual needs. This self-awareness is central when determining competence and learning needs.

Learning activity 2.4 Strengths, Weaknesses, Opportunities and Threats (SWOT)

Think about your own levels of competency: what you are good at , what you are less good at, what you would like to know more about, what you need to know more about, and the possible consequences of knowing or not knowing.

Think about all these things and try to put them in the SWOT table below.

Strengths	Weaknesses
Opportunities	Threats

Once you have done this, think about your weaknesses and identify your number one priority – the area of competence you need to improve most urgently.

Then develop an action plan (with your line manager or mentor) to ensure that you can work towards meeting that need.

Competence in nursing is not static. Although an individual may attain competence in one area of practice, that area of practice is likely to evolve and change with the individual's own developing experience, in which their perceived levels of competence will shift over time. This is illustrated in the early work of Benner (1984) who conceptualised the journey of an individual nurse from novice to expert through five stages of practice:

1. Novice
2. Advanced beginner
3. Competent
4. Proficient
5. Expert.

These stages can be experienced in several different ways. Firstly, the 'journey' may be a straight linear progression from stage 1 (novice) to stage 5 (expert). However, more frequently, an individual is likely to be at different stages for different elements of their role, progressing upwards in some areas more rapidly than others. As new elements are added to their role, or their role develops and progresses consistently adding in new elements, an individual nurse may find themselves back at the earlier stages for some role elements and may never attain expert levels of competence in all areas of their work.

The inherent difficulty of determining competence, and the ever-changing nature of nursing competence, has led to the development of several different approaches by which it can be measured across the whole spectrum of nursing practice. These are commonly articulated when focusing on education and pre-qualifying nursing practice.

For qualified nurses, determining competency is much more complex and, apart from generic assumptions about professional competence, this has led to the development of specific clinical competencies in many specialised areas of practice, as well as the development of a range of bespoke tools designed to test differing aspects of this competence. The legitimacy of these varied competency benchmarks and measures is subject to debate. Responsibility for the validity and currency of any competency guidelines is complex and lies in several places: the individual nurse who is responsible for self-assessment of their own competencies; the employer and their expectations of the nurse's role and the mechanisms they have put in place to monitor competency; and finally the professional regulatory body.

When considering competency, it is also important to recognise that the values of the professional, both individually and collectively, for what can be considered competent practice, may not always be the same as the values of those experiencing and using nursing care. Although it is extremely important for nurses to employ both self-regulation and professional regulation to maintain and develop their own standards of competence, it is equally important for nurses not to lose sight of the needs and experiences of the individuals using nursing services. It is clear from the literature that there is some divergence between patients' and professionals' views of nursing competence which cannot be ignored. (Think about what you may have learned about this divergence in Learning activity 2.2 above.)

When asked, patients have consistently identified a limited number of expectations of competent nurses:

- Knowledge of different conditions
- Knowledge of treatment of different conditions
- Knowledge of symptoms of different conditions
- Ability to provide advice or signposting
- Need to recognise patients' own expert knowledge
- Need to treat individuals with respect
- Ability to work collaboratively.

(Taken from Erwin et al. 2017, Kiljunen et al. 2017)

Competence in nursing practice is complex and difficult to define, but competence is the firm responsibility of the individual nurse, in collaboration with the standards and guidance of their employer and their professional body. Every person making use of nursing care across all the areas of nursing practice has a clear right to expect competent practice. Great nurses must recognise that competence is not static, but dynamic and ever-changing. Only through a process of constant self-appraisal can competence be maintained. Aside from their personal competence, as professional registrants, nurses must also be constantly aware of the practices of others and their professional responsibly to protect the public by maintaining, developing and enforcing high levels of competent care wherever they practise. The development of higher levels of competence is an ongoing task for both the individual and the profession but it is integral to ensuring that users of nursing care receive the standards of practice they have a right to expect. Further consideration will be given to developing skills and competence in Chapter 4.

Personal integrity and professional conduct

It is evident that autonomy and taking personal responsibility for your actions is a vital element of being a great nurse. This autonomous responsibility can be encapsulated by the idea of 'personal integrity'.

The American Nurses Association (2015) defines integrity as an individual's internal quality which can be recognised by others as honesty and moral consistency. High levels of personal integrity have long been considered essential to the nursing profession, with the integrity of nurses rated consistently as high in several polls of members of the public. If nurses lack personal integrity, their ability to fulfil public expectations of their role is seriously compromised; it is also likely that their actions will be contrary to the values of the profession, resulting in poor, if not negligent, standards of practice.

The concept of personal integrity is both complex and multifaceted and, in order to fully demonstrate integrity of practice, the following elements should be considered:

- Trust
- Honesty
- Competency
- Ethical behaviour

- Professionalism
- Safety
- Accountability.

(Taken from: Schmidt & McArthur 2018, Devine & Chin 2018, Sellman 2011)

Although, when considering integrity, there is a great deal of emphasis on personal responsibility for one's own actions, there is also recognition that, in some situations, integrity may encompass more than one individual and there is a shared collective responsibility. This is particularly relevant in nursing practice, with its emphasis on working collaboratively within multidisciplinary teams for the benefit of patient care. The ability of the team to demonstrate integrity is likely to be influenced by the culture of the workplace, its leadership and the environment in which the individual is placed.

A collective approach to integrity can be positive, supporting the individual to take personal responsibility for their own actions, as well as holding them responsible for any lapses or failings in care. However, collective responsibility can also lead to more negative consequences if benchmarks of practice are set low, with a culture of complacency, lack of accountability or individuals being disempowered and feeling unable to exercise their own personal integrity (see Chapter 1, Box 1.4).

There may also be occasions when there is a conflict between the personal integrity of the individual and the professional integrity required by their role. For instance, a nurse may make a personal decision not to have a vaccination. However, if they then contract the disease in question, there is a conflict with their professional integrity which requires them to ensure that they are fit to practise. To add further complexity, a nurse may personally decide not to smoke or drink alcohol during pregnancy but then be required to work with people whose views and actions are different, leading to compromise between the individual's personal integrity and the integrity required of their professional role.

Finding a balance between personal and professional integrity can be difficult, and not all aspects of personal integrity can be internalised into professional practice or vice versa. When becoming a great nurse, recognition of this conundrum is vital, as standards of personal integrity are the foundation of all core values.

Personal integrity is closely linked to professional conduct. In the UK this is regulated by the Nursing and Midwifery Council (NMC) and standards are set out in *The Code* (2018) (see Chapter 1, Table 1.2): which:

> 'sets out common standards of conduct and behaviour for those on our register. This provides a clear, consistent and positive message to patients, service users and colleagues about what they can expect of those who provide nursing or midwifery care.'

There is considerable overlap between the requirements of *The Code* and the core values expected of a great nurse but, importantly, failure to adhere to the regulatory body's *Code* can result in disciplinary action and removal from the professional register.

Professional conduct is also closely linked to personal conduct and, as with integrity, nurses need to act in accordance with the expectations of their professional code, which covers all aspects of their lives. Consequently, personal conduct is an all-encompassing concept by which great nurses must demonstrate integrity, positive role modelling and professional behaviour at all times in order to maintain the trust and respect of those needing nursing care, and not damage the reputation of the profession. It is striking that professional conduct is most remarked upon when it is absent, either through direct failings in care or through personal conduct that is considered inappropriate for holders of this highly regarded professional role.

Professional conduct investigations into nursing in the UK focus on six main areas:

- Misconduct (including clinical misconduct)
- Lack of competence
- Criminal convictions
- Serious ill health
- Not having the necessary knowledge of the English language
- Fraudulent access to the register.

There are similar key concerns across the international arena of nursing practice, wherever the profession has an accountable, regulatory body. However, it is important to keep this in perspective: within the UK, the NMC (2017) routinely reports that fewer than 1% of the nearly 700,000 qualified nurse registrants have any concerns raised about them.

Personal integrity and professional conduct are clearly closely interrelated concepts that underpin all core values in nursing. To become a great nurse, it is imperative that a nurse understand how complex integrity is, to be clear about their own personal and professional standards, and to be able to role model best practice when both on and off duty, safeguarding the reputation of the profession in order to maintain public trust and respect.

Valuing self – the labour of nursing and the need for self-respect and self-caring

The core nursing values outlined above do not include one other essential attribute of great nursing – and this is the 'labour' of nursing, and the values that underpin individual nurses' own self-respect and self-caring attributes.

Much of this book is about compassion and caring. When compassion is described in relation to nursing, the definitions often highlight the nurse's attitude towards others and how this is demonstrated by their actions and behaviour. However, Gilbert (2010, p. xiii) talks about compassion for 'self'; he says:

'Compassion can be defined in many ways, but its essence is a basic kindness, with a deep awareness of the suffering of oneself and of other living things'.

He sees 'self-compassion' as an important process for dealing with life's problems.

Caring for others is associated with an emotional component that goes beyond simply undertaking physical or technical tasks. As mentioned previously, nurses are expected to engage emotionally with their work and use of the 'Heart' is an important component of being a 'good nurse'. This is often referred to as the 'emotional labour' of nursing (Smith 2012) because so much is expected of nurses' conduct and behaviour, and nurses' work can be both physically and emotionally challenging. It is traditional for nurses to be regarded as 'selfless', even in modern times. This encourages nurses not to practise self-care, which then has an impact on patient care because the nurse is not able to perform to a high standard. It's important for nurses to recognise this, and learn to care for themselves in order to prevent the challenges becoming too much and affecting their work negatively. It is not easy to carry out self-care and this issue is discussed a great deal within the nursing community, yet there are many nurses who still do not manage to look after their own needs.

Stress and burnout commonly affect nurses and other healthcare professionals. Working under pressure with limited resources, in emotionally charged situations in which others are suffering, requires great strength of character and empathy. These demands can have a detrimental impact on nurses and they can end up suffering from 'compassion fatigue' with a resultant impact on both quality of care and the wellbeing of the nurse. In such circumstances, self-compassion is an important protective mechanism.

This problem has been studied by researchers such as Duarte *et al.* (2016, p. 1) who summarise their work by stating that:

> '... self-compassion and self-care skills, i.e., a tendency to be kind and understanding toward oneself, to feel interconnected with other people and to hold negative experiences with mindful awareness, may be an important feature in nursing educational interventions that aim to reduce burnout and compassion fatigue...'

The next two learning activities are designed to help you to think about the importance of self-care and the emotional labour which underpins being a great nurse. They will also enable you to shift the focus to how great nurses can start to work towards addressing both their own and others' self-care needs.

Learning activity 2.5 Self-care

There are several elements of the summary provided by Duarte et al. (2016) that are worth thinking about in more detail. Look at the quotation again and consider the following questions:

What does the above quotation suggest that you could do, as an individual nurse, to develop your 'self-care' skills and capacity?

What do you think would be involved in being 'kind and understanding' towards yourself?

What does it mean to 'hold negative experiences with mindful awareness'?

Think about when you have had a 'bad day' – an emotionally and/or physically draining one – be it as a nurse or in some other aspect of life.

What did you do (or what could you have done) to help you deal with that experience in a self-caring way?

Learning activity 2.6 Scenario – self-compassion

You have just started working in a new clinical area. It is a very demanding and busy clinical setting with very high workloads, and at the end of most days you are both physically and emotionally exhausted. It seems to be the culture here to work flat-out, without breaks, and the staff members do not even have time to talk to each other when something distressing has happened. You are worried that you are not going to be able to sustain this pattern of work for very long, even though you enjoy the patient activity and contact it gives you and it is what you have always wanted to do.

Place yourself in this imaginary situation (although, for many nurses, this is a reality). Ask yourself the following questions:

- What can I do to take care of myself more self-compassionately in this situation?
- Who else could I involve in a plan for self-care and how might I approach them?
- How could I approach the other staff members to talk about this issue?

Conclusion

Being a great nurse is not easy but thoughtful consideration of the core values which underpin all aspects of nursing practice provides individual nurses with an essential framework to support best-quality practice. These values should be internalised into personal professional practice and form the basis for reflection and ongoing personal development.

The key points from this chapter can best be summarised in six key steps, which are essential for all great nurses – see Box 2.3 below.

Box 2.3 How to be a great nurse – six core values

1. Be kind to others and sensitive to each individual's needs
2. Remember that dignity and respect are central to everything you do
3. Set aside your own judgements to focus on the individual
4. Competence in nursing practice requires constant self-appraisal
5. Clarify your own personal and professional standards of integrity
6. Pay attention to your own need for self-care.

Recommendations for further study

Baillie, L. & Black, S. (2015). *Professional values in nursing*. Boca Raton: CRC Press.

McSherry, W., McSherry, R. & Watson, R. (2012). *Care in nursing. Principles, values and skills*. Oxford: Oxford University Press.

Sellman, D. (2011). *What makes a good nurse: Why the virtues are important for nurses*. London: Jessica Kingsley.

Smith, P. (2012). *The emotional labour of nursing revisited. Can nurses still care?* 2nd edn. Houndmills: Palgrave Macmillan.

References

Adams, K.L. & Iseler J.I. (2014). The relationship of bedside nurses' emotional intelligence with quality of care. *Journal of Nursing Care Quality*. **29**(2), 174–181.

Allen, J. & Dennis, M. (2009). Dignity and respect matter. *British Journal of Healthcare Assistants*. **3**, 594–98.

American Association of Colleges of Nursing (2008). *The essentials of baccalaureate education for professional nursing practice.* https://www.aacnnursing.org/Education-Resources/AACN-Essentials (last accessed 10.1.2020).

American Nurses Association (2015). *The Code of Ethics for Nurses with interpretative statements.* https://www.nursingworld.org/practice-policy/nursing-excellence/ethics/code-of-ethics-for-nurses/ (last accessed 10.1.2020).

Beauvais, A.M., Brady, N., O'Shea, E.R. & Griffin, M.T.Q. (2011). Emotional intelligence and nursing performance among nursing students. *Nursing Faculty Publications*. **17**.

Benner, P. (1984). *From novice to expert: Excellence and power in clinical nursing practice.* Menlo Park, CA: Addison-Wesley.

Census (2010). https://www.census.gov/newsroom/releases/archives/2010_census/cb11-cn125.html (last accessed 11.1.2020).

Clark, J. (2010). Defining the concept of dignity and developing a model to promote its use in practice. *Nursing Times*. **106**, 20.

Department of Health (2012). *Transforming care: A national response to Winterbourne View Hospital, Department of Health Review, Final Report.* https://www.gov.uk/government/uploads/system/uploads/attachment_data/file/213215/final-report.pdf (last accessed 11.1.2020).

Devine, C.A. & Chin, E.D. (2018). Integrity in nursing students: A concept analysis. *Nurse Education Today*. **60**, 133–38.

Doyle, K., Hungerford, C. & Cruickshank, M. (2014). Reviewing tribunal cases and nurse behaviour: putting empathy back into nurse education with Bloom's taxonomy. *Nurse Education Today*. **34**, 1069–73.

Duarte, J., Pinto-Goureia, J. & Cruz, B. (2016). Relationship between nurses' empathy, self-compassion and dimensions of professional quality of life: a cross sectional study. *International Journal of Nursing Studies*. **60**, 1–11.

Erwin, J., Edwards, K., Woolf, A., Whitcombe, S. & Kilty, S. (2017). Better arthritis care: patients' expectations and priorities, the competencies that community-based health professionals need to improve their care of people with arthritis? *Musculoskeletal Care*. **16**, 60–66.

Ethnicity facts and figures (2018). *Ethnicity facts and figures.* https://www.ethnicity-facts-figures.service.gov.uk/ (last accessed 11.1.2020).

Francis, R. (2010). *Independent inquiry into care provided by Mid Staffordshire NHS Foundation Trust January 2005–March 2009.* http://webarchive.nationalarchives.gov.uk/20150407084003/http://www.midstaffspublicinquiry.com/key-documents (last accessed 11.1.2020).

Francis, R. (2013). *The Mid Staffordshire NHS Foundation Trust Public Inquiry* http://webarchive.nationalarchives.gov.uk/20150407084003/http://www.midstaffspublicinquiry.com/ (last accessed 11.1.2020).

Gilbert, P. (2010). An introduction to compassion focused therapy in cognitive behavioural therapy. *International Journal of Cognitive Therapy*. **3**, 97–112.

International Council of Nurses (ICN) (2012). *The ICN Code of Ethics for Nurses.* Geneva, Switzerland: ICN.

Kiljunen, O., Kankkunen, P., Partanen, P. & Valimaki, T. (2017). Family members' expectations regarding nurses' competence in care homes: a qualitative interview study. *Scandinavian Journal of the Caring Sciences*. **32**, 1018–26.

Kovner, C.T., Djukic, M., Jun, J., Fletcher, F., Fatehi, F.K. & Brewer, C.S. (2018). Diversity and education of the nursing workforce 2006–2016. *Nursing Outlook*. **66**, 160–67.

Larsson, G., Widmark, V, Lampic, C., Von Essen, L. & Sjoden, P.O. (1998). Cancer patient and staff ratings of the importance of caring behaviours and their relations to patient anxiety and depression. *Journal of Advanced Nursing*. **27**, 855–64.

Lowe, J. & Archibald, C. (2009). Cultural diversity: the intention of nursing. *Nursing Forum*. **44**(1), 11–18.

Mackintosh, C. (2000). Is there a place for 'care' within nursing? *International Journal of Nursing Studies*. **37**(4), 321–27.

Maslach, C., Schafeli, E.B. & Leiter, M.P. (2001). Job burnout. *Annual Review of Psychology*. **52**, 397–422.

Moore, H.A. & Gaviola, M.S. (2018). Engaging students in a culture of integrity. *Journal of Nursing Education*. **57**(4), 237–39.

National League for Nurses (NLN) (2018). *Core values*. http://www.nln.org/about/core-values (last accessed 11.1.2020).

National Nursing Research Unit (NNRU) (2009). *Nursing competence: what are we assessing and how should it be measured?* King's College London. https://www.kcl.ac.uk/nmpc/research/nnru/policy/policy-plus-issues-by-theme/boundaries-regulation-competence/policyissue18.pdf (last accessed 11.1.2020).

NHS England (2018). *The 6 Cs*. https://www.england.nhs.uk/6cs/wp-content/uploads/sites/25/2015/03/introducing-the-6cs.pdf (last accessed 11.1.2020).

Nursing and Midwifery Council (NMC) (2015). *The Code*. https://www.nmc.org.uk/globalassets/sitedocuments/nmc-publications/nmc-code.pdf (last accessed 11.1.2020).

Nursing and Midwifery Council (NMC) (2017). *Annual Fitness to Practise Report 2016–17*. https://www.nmc.org.uk/globalassets/sitedocuments/annual_reports_and_accounts/ftpannualreports/annual-fitness-to-practise-report-2016-2017.pdf (last accessed 11.1.2020).

NMC (2018) *Part 1: Standards framework for nursing and midwifery education*. https://www.nmc.org.uk/standards-for-education-and-training/standards-framework-for-nursing-and-midwifery-education/ (last accessed 11.1.2020).

Nursing and Midwifery Council (NMC) (2018). *The Code*. https://www.nmc.org.uk/globalassets/sitedocuments/nmc-publications/nmc-code.pdf (last accessed 11.1.2020).

Nursing and Midwifery Council (NMC) (2019). *Future nurse: Standards of proficiency for registered nurses*. https://www.nmc.org.uk/globalassets/sitedocuments/education-standards/future-nurse-proficiencies.pdf (last accessed 11.1.2020).

Patients Association (2020). https://www.patients-association.org.uk/ (last accessed 11.1.2020).

Rankin, B. (2013). Emotional intelligence: enhancing values-based practice and compassionate care in nursing. *Journal of Advanced Nursing*. **69**, 12.

Royal College of Nursing (RCN) (2016). *Preserving people's dignity*. https://rcni.com/hosted-content/rcn/first-steps/preserving-peoples-dignity (last accessed 11.1.2020).

Royal College of Nursing (RCN) (2018). *Principles of nursing practice*. https://www.rcn.org.uk/professional-development/principles-of-nursing-practice (last accessed 11.1.2020).

Schmidt, B.J. & McArthur, E.C. (2018). Professional nursing values: A concept analysis. *Nursing Forum*. **53**, 69–75.

Sellman, D. (2011). *What makes a good nurse: Why the virtues are important for nurses*. London: Jessica Kingsley.

Smith, P. (2012). *The emotional labour of nursing revisited. Can nurses still care?* 2nd edn. Houndmills: Palgrave Macmillan.

Smith, K.B., Profetto-McGrath, J., & Cummings, G.G. (2009). Emotional intelligence and nursing: an integrative literature review. *International Journal of Nursing Studies*. **46**, 1624–36.

Winship, G. (2010). Is emotional intelligence an important concept for nursing practice? *Journal of Psychiatric and Mental Health Nursing*. **17**, 940–48.

Zangaro, G.A., Streeter, R. & Li, T. (2018). Trends in racial and ethnic demographics of the nursing workforce; 2000–2015. *Nursing Outlook*. **66**, 365–71.

Chapter 3

Learning to be a great nurse

Introduction

Learning is an integral part of becoming a great nurse. Great nurses are not born great and, although some people may have innate personality traits which make them naturally predisposed towards the nursing profession, good nurses only become really great at what they do if they have an ongoing commitment to lifelong learning.

Great nurses usually start their learning journey long before they join the nursing profession, observing and participating in the care of family members or friends, learning from their own experiences and those of others, and feeding their own natural curiosity to know more, to understand the reasons why, and to work out how things can be done in the best possible way. This urge to know is complemented by formal education (at school, at college and at university), and all these elements combine to shape the individual, to feed the need for knowledge, and to deepen and broaden their understanding of what makes nurses great.

This chapter will consider the main elements of the learning process that help nurses to become great by using the Head, Heart and Hand.

Learning

The way people actually learn is hotly debated. There are several different ideas about learning which are now commonly accepted and these are best classified as being based on three key theories:

- The stimulus–response theory
- Cognitive theories
- Humanistic theories.

The stimulus–response theory (which is also linked to behaviourism) encapsulates several broad ideas, including those based on what is known as 'conditioning' (someone learning to behave in a certain way in response to a learnt stimulus). It also includes the idea of learning as a consequence of trial and error or experimentation. This type of learning is commonly seen in young children and animals – for example, a young child learning not to touch something which is hot, as they will be burnt. Stimulus–response learning can also involve role modelling the behaviour of others; again, someone may see the way someone else behaves in a certain situation and mimic that behaviour. If that behaviour gains praise, or some other form of reward, the person learns that this is a positive thing to do and the behaviour is reinforced.

Cognitive theories of learning focus on how people think about certain things; so, rather than breaking down learning into the more concrete form demanded by the stimulus–response theory, cognitive theories suggest that people learn by putting ideas together as a process of assimilation or concept-forming. Cognitive theorists also talk about learning as a process of discovery or information processing; putting ideas and knowledge together to form something new and then making a judgement about how useful that new knowledge is, and whether and where it can be applied.

Humanistic theories are wide-ranging and attempt to combine elements of learning that are overlooked in the other two theories. These include important individual learning components such as feelings and experiences which may be related to personal attitudes and values. Humanistic learning theories focus on ideas such as self-actualisation; this approach to education is frequently student-centred with an emphasis on how the 'teacher' can support the learner, the personal needs of the learner and the individual meaning of the learning experience.

It is beyond the scope of this book to consider these theories in depth but, if you would like to know more, there is a range of further reading on this subject listed at the end of this chapter. It is important to recognise that all these learning theories support the fundamental idea that learning takes place in many ways and there is no one 'correct' way to learn.

Just as there are several theories about how people learn, there are also several ways in which learners can be categorised. The best-known ways of categorising learners focus on different types of 'learning styles' that people may have a preference for, and this has resulted in a number of different ways in which learning styles can be identified. One of the most commonly used is the 'Seven Learning Styles' classification system below.

Box 3.1 The seven learning styles

- Visual (spatial): The learner prefers using pictures, images and spatial understanding
- Aural (auditory-musical): The learner prefers using sound and music
- Verbal (linguistic): The learner prefers using words, both in speech and writing
- Physical (kinaesthetic): The learner prefers using their body, hands and sense of touch
- Logical (mathematical): The learner prefers using logic, reasoning and systems
- Social (interpersonal): The learner prefers to learn in groups or with other people
- Solitary (intrapersonal): The learner prefers to work alone and use self-study

From: https://www.learning-styles-online.com/overview/

A more complex way of explaining learning styles was developed by Honey and Mumford (1986), building on the earlier work of Kolb (1976). They used Kolb's idea of four different types of learners, Activists, Reflectors, Theorists and Pragmatists, and adapted this into a cycle of learning which moves through the stages of: concrete experience, reflective observation, abstract conceptualisation and active experimentation. In this cycle, the individual learner may also be more inclined towards one or the other of these stages by their positioning on two related continuums – those of perception and processing (see Figure 3.1).

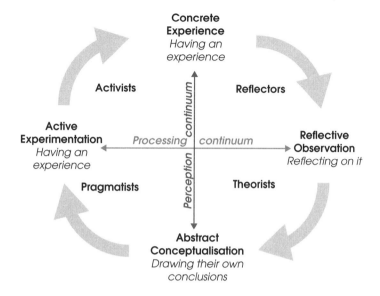

Figure 3.1 Honey and Mumford (1986) model of learning styles

Work on individual learning styles has been further developed into several self-administered tests, collectively known as learning inventories, which allow an individual to work out which type of learning style best suits their learning needs. Knowing which type of learning style works best for each individual can be valuable for the learner, and also when developing a learning programme and undertaking activities such as mentorship and preceptorship which will be discussed later in this chapter.

Learning activity 3.1 Your learning style

Think about yourself and your own personal learning style:

- In the past, what type of learning has really worked for you?
- Where and how have you learned the most?

Have a look at Honey and Mumford's Learning Style Inventory in the appendix of this book. It takes around 10–15 minutes to complete. See if the tool suggests which learning style is the best for you. Now you have an idea about what type of learning style works best for you, how can you use that to make the best use of future learning opportunities?

Lifelong learning in nursing

Having an understanding of how we and others learn is essential when considering the importance of lifelong learning. The benefits of lifelong learning across the whole population are widely recognised, with both direct and indirect effects. Direct effects are those derived directly from a course of study, be it a study-day or a formal educational programme. Indirect effects are often unintended and frequently unique to the individual. They may include important personal attributes (such as increased self-confidence and better career prospects) as well as a range of potential benefits to others, including family members, the community and employers.

The direct and indirect benefits of lifelong learning can be applied directly to great nurses using both the Head and the Hand. Imagine, for example, that you are a nurse working with patients who smoke and have recently attended a study day on smoking cessation. Your knowledge of how to support someone in giving up smoking can be applied directly to your work role; it may help your patients, but you may also be able to directly help other members of staff, your family members and friends. Your personal confidence in providing support in this area will also increase. Your support of patients may result in them reducing or giving up smoking and this will have direct positive consequences for them, as well as indirect consequences for their friends and families, who may now be able to live in a smoke-free environment, or live with someone who is less likely to suffer from the health consequences of long-term smoking and who can serve as a positive role model on how to give up.

Within healthcare, the overall benefits for lifelong learning have been clearly identified, and these can be summarised in five principles (see Box 3.2).

Box 3.2 Principles of lifelong learning

1. Lifelong learning is each person's responsibility in negotiation with their employer.
2. Lifelong learning should be of benefit to those using healthcare services.
3. Lifelong learning should help improve the quality of service delivery.
4. Lifelong learning should be relevant to each person's area of practice.
5. Lifelong learning and any impact should be recorded.

(Taken from: The Interprofessional CPD and Lifelong Learning UK Working Group 2019)

Lifelong learning is, therefore, fundamental to great nursing care. It is important to note that this is not just about attending courses or study days. Learning can take place anywhere and at any time and take numerous forms. Spencer (2009) argues that one of the most important attributes a nurse can have, which supports lifelong learning, is the urge to be curious, to ask questions about what nurses do and why they do it and then to seek the answers.

The importance of lifelong learning in great nursing practice is reflected in the way it has been incorporated in professional nursing standards. The International Council of Nurses (2010) states that nurses must undertake 'a life-long process of maintaining and enhancing the competencies of the nurse'. In the UK, the NMC *Code* (2018) clearly states (in Section 6.2) that all nurses have an obligation to 'Maintain the knowledge and skills you need for safe and effective practice.'

This is further encapsulated in the NMC standards for Pre-Registration Nursing Programmes (2018c) and in the NMC Standards of Proficiency for Registered Nurses (2018a) in which all nurses must: 'take responsibility for continuous self-reflection, seeking and responding to support and feedback to develop their professional knowledge and skills'.

Evidence of a minimum of 35 hours of continuous professional development (CPD), which can be considered as part of this lifelong learning, is now required in the three-yearly revalidation process developed by the NMC for all registered nurses in the UK who wish to remain on the professional register (NMC 2016).

Learning activity 3.2 Planning learning

When thinking about your own learning, consider what you are currently curious to know more about.

Once you have identified something, try the following steps:

1. How ready are you to learn something new? Do you have the time, the resources and the commitment?
2. If you are ready to learn, what do you intend to learn? What are your goals? Do you want formal study or something more self-directed?
3. Once you have established your goals, you need to undertake the actual learning, be this reading, talking to colleagues, attending a study day or enrolling on a course.
4. Finally, you need to evaluate what you have learned. Have you learned enough? Was it useful? How can you use it in the future?

From this brief discussion of the essential nature of lifelong learning within nursing, it is clear that responsibility for maintaining this learning lies primarily with the individual nurse. Nurses may be held accountable by their professional bodies and employers for failure to uphold professional standards, but responsibility for ensuring that the standards for lifelong learning are met is firmly with the individual. Consequently, great nurses must also be self-directed, committed and motivated to learn. The central importance of the individual nurse's commitment to this is best encapsulated diagrammatically in the NMC (2014) *Standards for Competence for Registered Nurses*. Clearly, self-directed learning, in theory and practice, is essential to achieve competence in all areas and fields of nursing practice (see Figure 3.2).

Commitment to lifelong learning, with its emphasis on Hand and Head, is essential for all great nurses, regardless of their position in the organisational structure or how many years' experience they possess. It is also well-recognised that nursing can be a stressful and demanding profession, and the need to continually keep updated can be seen as an additional burden by many staff, rather than an integral component of great nursing practice. The development of a healthcare culture that supports lifelong learning in nursing is essential in order to support individual nurses to foster their curiosity, improve their practice and maintain their personal motivation and commitment.

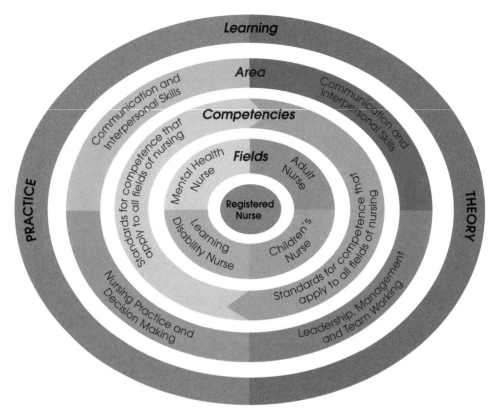

Figure 3.2 NMC (2014) Standards for Competence for Registered Nurses

Learning from others

So far in this chapter the focus has been on the individual nurse and their personal responsibility for lifelong learning. However, much of this lifelong learning does not take place in isolation, nurses routinely work in multidisciplinary healthcare teams and much of the lifelong learning needed to become a great nurse can be gained through the direct and indirect support of others. Pre-registration student nurses, at both undergraduate and postgraduate levels of study, are generally considered to be neophytes or beginners in learning the skills needed to become a great nurse. To facilitate their own learning, they can rely on the support of many others, including university lecturers, resources and support services, mentors in clinical practice, peers and family and friends. Once qualified, nurses may no longer have the formal support of an academic institution, but can continue to access educational support opportunities from their professional body, their employer, a preceptorship programme, peer support and family and friends, as well as a range of CPD learning opportunities.

Mentorship

A mentor is one of the best-known international terms to identify someone whose role is specifically to support learning – in this context, normally in pre-registration student nurse education. Mentorship can be a formal role identified by an employer as forming part of someone's role description, and can involve the mentor in formal training in preparation to undertake the role and the assessment which is normally part of it.

Mentors are vital in providing students with the support and guidance they need during placement learning, and as role models of best practice and positive professional values. They have a formal role in observing students' practice (providing feedback on their competence, and their ability to integrate theory with the practice they are involved in) and formally assessing a student's practice-related learning outcomes (Royal College of Nursing 2017).

Until recently, formal training recognised by the NMC was an essential requirement for anyone undertaking the mentorship role in the UK. This has recently been revised and, from 2019 onwards, the requirement for formal training will no longer exist. Instead, mentors will be replaced by practice assessors and practice supervisors. Practice assessors will assess and confirm a student's achievements in practice, while practice supervisors will provide direct hands-on supervision. These roles may be undertaken by any registered nurse and can also be carried out by other registered health and social care professionals (NMC 2018b).

Preceptorship

Preceptorship is another well-recognised role for supporting nurses in lifelong learning. The main difference from mentorship is that a preceptor focuses on newly qualified nursing staff and the transition from the role of student to fully qualified member of staff. The input of preceptors may also be required when nurses transfer from one clinical specialist area to another, change employment to a different clinical setting, develop a new set of skills or undertake a specific clinical CPD activity.

Periods of preceptorship may vary across organisations, and the nature of the relationship can range from very formal to a much more relaxed 'buddy' relationship. There are real benefits, however, to the use of preceptors and preceptorship transitions for all nurses and these have been widely recognised as:

- Supporting new staff orientation into a new organisation
- Improving recruitment and retention in a clinical area
- Reducing staff sickness absence
- Increasing staff satisfaction
- Supporting the development of more confident skilled staff.

(Taken from: New Zealand Nurse Educators Preceptorship Subgroup 2010)

Clinical supervision

Lifelong learning can also be supported by those working as supervisors. The term 'supervision' can be interpreted in several ways; in the UK, the new practice supervisor role for pre-registration nursing students is a formal managerial approach, or a means of enhancing clinical/professional practice across a range of healthcare professions. Within nursing and healthcare globally, the term clinical supervision is most frequently used and is usually considered to be separate from formal managerial supervision, which is carried out by a line manager.

According to the Care Quality Commission (2013), clinical supervision is designed to:

'...provide a safe and confidential environment for staff to reflect on and discuss their work, and their personal and professional responses to their work. The focus is on supporting staff in their personal and professional development and in reflecting on their practice...'

Successful clinical supervision has been recognised as achieving several benefits for the individual, the organisation and service users. According to Koivu *et al.* 2012, the Care Quality Commission 2013, and Bifarin and Stonehouse 2017, it offers the individual:

- Improved job satisfaction
- Increased knowledge
- Reduced emotional stress and burnout
- Improved self-confidence.

For the organisation, it provides:

- Improved job satisfaction
- Improved retention of staff and reduced staff turnover
- Improved staff effectiveness
- Good clinical governance.

For service users, it:

- Helps ensure they receive the best-quality care from well-supported staff.

In the UK, although there is no formal regulatory requirement for qualified nurses to receive regular clinical supervision (although there *are* for midwives), the use of clinical supervision is considered to be good practice and, although not explicit, can be implied in many areas of the NMC *Code* (2018), including Section 8.4: 'Work with colleagues to evaluate the quality of your work and that of the team'.

Clinical supervision can take place in several ways: as one-to-one in a supervisor–supervisee relationship, as part of group supervision with a small group of practitioners and a supervisor, and in the form of peer clinical supervision where practitioners are of an equal standing and learn from each other.

Despite the recognised benefits of clinical supervision, it is not used as widely as it could be within nursing practice in the UK. There is often confusion over the roles of supervisor and supervisee, and between clinical supervision and more formal managerial supervision. The lack of a regulatory requirement for clinical supervision among qualified nursing staff can mean that some employing organisations are less supportive of this approach. There may therefore be limited formal encouragement to undertake clinical supervision, resulting in few resources, and the prioritising of other activities, leading to a culture that places little importance on this type of activity.

Role modelling

A less formal, but equally valuable, approach to lifelong learning is the use of positive role models as a vital learning resource. The Stimulus–Response model of learning (see p. 35) places its main emphasis on learning that takes place from the earliest age, based on the individual observing and copying what others do. Consequently, learning from role models is an innate skill that we all possess. It is important to note that role modelling can have both positive and negative impacts, depending on the chosen role model. For example, a young child may learn poor habits from role models just as easily as learning good ones, and this is equally relevant to the use of role models in professional nursing practice.

The use of role models in lifelong learning is considered to be most significant in the learning that takes place when a more junior member of staff observes and learns from a more senior member of staff who is considered to be 'good at their job'. This is partly encapsulated by the idea common to mentorship, preceptorship and clinical supervision – that a student or more junior member of staff learns from a more experienced person who can also act as a role model of good practice. However, this does not have to be hierarchical and anyone can be a role model. Everyone, regardless of experience or seniority, can continue to learn by observing others.

The key to successful lifelong learning through role modelling is the discrimination required to identify positive professional role models (Felstead & Springett 2014). Over the course of their undergraduate education programme and subsequent career, nurses are exposed to many and varied role models, some of whom will have more positive attributes than others and it is unlikely that a nurse will find one individual who is their ideal role model. Instead, learning from role modelling is likely to be a patchwork, acquiring a range of skills, values and attitudes from a wide range of exposures that require the individual to recognise the positive attributes of colleagues they would aspire to be like, and to reject learning from the more negative role models they encounter. To summarise, effective learning from role models involves working towards becoming a 'great nurse' and moving away from becoming the type of nurse 'you don't want to be'.

Learning activity 3.3 Role modelling

As role modelling is an important part of learning, it is useful to think back on your own learning process and the people you have come across who you have seen as positive role models.

- Try to identify who those people were. What made them stand out in your own mind as a positive role model?
- What do you feel you learned from each of them?
- Because there may be several people, how about writing a list and then identifying what you learned from each of them?
- Thinking about your list, how have you included this learning in your current practice?
- Do you think you are now a really positive role model for others?
- How do you think you could become an even better role model?

Peer learning

Peer learning takes place when peers learn from each other, rather than within a more formal hierarchical structure such as a teacher–learner relationship. As with all types of learning from others, this can take place both informally (for example, in lecture room conversations), or more formally through a recognised process of peer-assisted learning and across a range of environments. Informal peer learning is like role modelling, in that it is an innate learning skill that individuals develop throughout their lifespan. When it takes place informally, learning from peers can capture the essential requirement of lifelong learning – to remain curious, to ask questions and to actively observe.

Because peer learning is an innate, ongoing process which is known to be beneficial, there have been several attempts to introduce it directly into the undergraduate nursing curriculum. This can be seen in the use of group or team task work and discussions, and also in educational schemes where more junior students are encouraged to learn from more senior ones (learning from 'near peers'). This can include clinical skills such as basic life support, and more theoretical elements of the programme, such as physiology, which students may struggle with. (To learn more about this, you could look at: Crawford & Cannon 2018, Nelwati & Chan 2018 and Irvine *et al.* 2018.)

Peer learning and near peer learning are effective ways of learning from others, not because of the expertise or experience of the participants (which may all be similar), but because it gives participants the opportunity to learn in what is generally considered to be a safe, supportive and judgement-free manner. As well as improving knowledge and skills, this can promote both self-confidence and self-directed learning. Although the more formal aspects of peer learning are currently seen most commonly in undergraduate programmes, its use as a form of clinical supervision (see above) is also considered beneficial for the development and maintenance of lifelong learning and is something all great nurses can use to their advantage.

Skills to learn from others

Learning from others can take place in many ways, some of which are discussed above. However, learning from others also requires certain qualities and skills. As lifelong learners, it is important that great nurses are:

- Prepared to take the initiative to learn
- Open to learning and new experiences
- Persistent in continuing to learn
- Receptive to feedback, both positive and negative
- Organised and self-disciplined
- Passionate about nursing and learning.

As a supporter of learning in others (be it as a mentor, preceptor, supervisor, role model or peer), it is also essential for a great nurse to be:

- Approachable and welcoming
- Supportive of learning
- Confident in their own skills and those of others
- Calm and reassuring
- Open to feedback, both positive and negative
- Passionate about nursing and learning.

Whatever the nature of the learning relationship, learning from others is a vital element in the lifelong learning process for all great nurses.

Learning from self

Reflective practice

Each day, nurses experience numerous events while giving patient care. Most of the time, they move on to the next event without thinking about the previous one. Sometimes these events are unsettling. Perhaps something didn't go as well as it should, the nurse experienced something new or something happened that was out of the ordinary, resulting in the type of emotional labour considered in Chapter 1. On these occasions, nurses often think more deeply about the event in a way that changes their practice in the future. Often, this happens automatically without any specific effort to do so. However, there are times when it is beneficial both for learning and for self-care, to deliberately follow a process to facilitate critical thought about the event and initiate change. This 'reflective practice' involves exploring experiences and/or feelings relating to an event or issue. This is a very individual process that is central to individual learning for every great nurse.

Dewey (1938) proposed that humans learn by doing and understanding the results of what they did. This is particularly true of nurses, simply because nursing is a profession that involves practical working with others. Kolb (1984) proposed that, following an experience, reflection was an important next step in being able to understand that experience and learn from it: in a sense, this is learning from self. In nursing, this 'reflective practice' is a process that uses experiences from practice as a catalyst for self-learning. By examining events, behaviours, thoughts and habits and developing new and extended knowledge, nurses can increase their expertise and provide care that is the best it can be. This process is central to bringing the 'head, heart and hand' elements of nursing together and being a great nurse. Self-reflection has been shown to stimulate practice learning, enhance the application of new knowledge and promote practice development. (To learn more about this, you might want to look at Miraglia & Asselin 2015.)

Schön (1983) describes the everyday experiences of nurses as seeming like life in the 'swampy lowlands', where the everyday world of work is messy and difficult, with problems and dilemmas that cannot always be solved by following rules or using established knowledge. Schön also proposed that there were two types of reflection:

● Reflection on action – contemplating events retrospectively

● Reflection in action – thinking about events as they occur rather than later.

Nurses are encouraged to record some of their reflections so that they can learn from them, discuss them with colleagues if they choose to do so, and develop them as evidence of their learning (e.g. in the UK, as part of the NMC revalidation process). Reflection is highly personal and individual, and the nurse must understand that they are not obliged to share this reflection with others, although discussing their experiences and thoughts with a colleague, peer or clinical supervisor can often be helpful.

At the beginning of their careers, when nurses are learning how to reflect effectively, they are often encouraged to use a reflective model as a guide to their reflection. Reflective models can help to structure this reflection and make it meaningful. There are several well-known models of reflection available that provide a structure for intentional reflection on practice.

Learning activity 3.4 Using a reflective model

Choosing a reflective model is a personal choice as to which works best for individual nurses, and no one model is better than any other. However, practitioners often continue to use the one they have always used, out of habit, without considering whether there may be something that suits them better.

- Undertake an internet search using terms such as 'reflection – model – nursing'
- Identify three models of reflection that you think sound interesting, which are different from the one you normally use.
- Consider the advantages and disadvantages of each model. Why would you prefer one to the other? Perhaps outline these in a table.
- Consider carefully which one of these you feel would be most likely to help you to be a great nurse. How would it help to develop the 'head, heart and hand' in your work?
- Experiment with this model and any other you thought might be useful to you by writing a reflection on the same event using the model/s you have chosen.

Being reflective

Reflection is meant to be challenging, so it is often difficult. It is important for nurses to believe in the value of reflection, and to actively participate. It encourages open-mindedness and enables practitioners to see things that they would not otherwise be so deeply aware of. Regular reflection enables nurses to actively learn throughout their careers and become great nurses. It helps to develop the self-awareness needed to be an emotionally intelligent practitioner who can work effectively using the 'head, heart and hand' approach. What matters is the ability to explore situations objectively and honestly, by writing in a way that enables expression of thoughts and feelings, as well as the application of theory and evidence. This takes practice of course, but it is not necessary for every reflection to be written perfectly; it simply needs to be understood by the individual nurse when they review it later.

Reflection after the event involves being able to remember what happened and what it felt like. For this reason, it is important to write the reflection as soon after the event as possible. It is also important that the reflection is clear and succinct. Writing too much can make reflection into a chore and reduce motivation. Sometimes reflection can raise more questions than answers, leading to a need to undertake further study as part of the lifelong learning process. Reflection can cause both personal and professional discomfort as well as resistance to change in both self and others.

Learning from evidence

Learning from self, and learning from others, as part of the lifelong learning process, are two vitally important ways for nurses to develop the skills of hand and head which are essential for the development of excellent standards of nursing knowledge and skills. However, they need to be used in conjunction with a third essential element, the use of literature and research-based evidence to underpin clinical practice and improve patient care. Learning from self, learning from others and learning from evidence all combine to support the hand and head of great nursing practice.

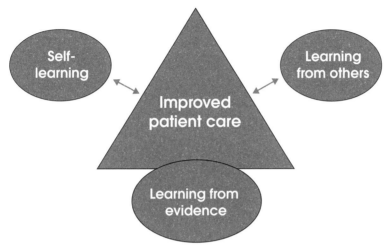

Figure 3.3 Lifelong learning to improve patient care

The idea of evidence-based practice was initially introduced to healthcare practice in the 1970s through the work of Archie Cochrane, an epidemiologist who recognised how difficult it was for practitioners to keep up to date with all the developments within their field. This meant that practice was largely carried out according to embedded, ritualised and outdated practices, with new evidence for improvements in practice undeveloped, ignored or unknown. Cochrane suggested that there was a need for readily available summaries of best practice as a quick access reference point for all healthcare professionals and this was the starting point for what is now known as evidence-based healthcare practice (Cochrane 1972).

From this starting point, the need for nurses to use evidence as a basis for much of their practice is now clearly recognised and, in the UK, the NMC (2018a) clearly states that in order for nurses to practise effectively they must 'Always practise in line with the best available evidence' (NMC 2018).

Whilst recognising the need for great nurses to include learning from evidence as part of their essential hand and heart skills, it is also important to consider what this 'evidence' consists of. The International Council of Nurses (2012) offers useful guidance in this area, describing evidence as: facts, which may be based on research findings or physiological principles, the expert experience of healthcare professionals and service users, and a range of individual attitudes and values, all of which may be balanced together to provide the best solution for each individual patient.

According to the Joanna Briggs Institute (2008), this can be summarised as:

'The combination of individual clinical or professional expertise with the best available external evidence to produce practice that is likely to lead to a positive outcome for a client or patient.'

The ICN (2012) suggests that learning from evidence should be seen as one part of a three-way relationship, which combines all elements of a patient experience to produce the best possible patient care outcomes.

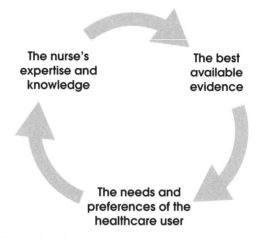

Figure 3.4 Elements of evidence-based practice

Evidence can take many forms, and it is important for nurses to be conscious of the need to be discerning when deciding what evidence to use, and to constantly make judgments about the respective values of the different evidence sources. This can change, depending on each situation or patient, and a particular evidence source may have differing value at different times.

Because evidence can come from many sources, great nurses sometimes need to develop a clear process for answering a particular clinical question they are interested in. This is most easily demonstrated when looking for evidence from published sources, such as academic research papers, where there is a recognised pathway for using literature/research-based evidence to support learning.

Looking for evidence usually involves:

● Identifying a clearly defined clinical question to be answered

● Breaking down that question into key elements

● Using these elements to carry out a systematic search of literature sources

● Determining the value of the evidence/information found

● Implementing actions based on findings from good-quality evidence sources.

Having a clearly defined question is an important first step. When using a systematic approach towards searching for evidence, it is also essential to have a clear focus. A question can take many forms. Commonly, nurses may want to know: 'what is the best treatment for X?', but equally it may be useful to compare one treatment with another: 'Does treatment X have better outcomes than treatment Y?'. However, asking a question may not be as simple as it first seems, as there are frequently issues with definitions and meanings. For example, Treatment X may have multiple names and therefore all variations of those names will need to be looked at. This difficulty is compounded when looking at best outcomes or best treatments. Definitions of what is 'best' vary considerably: is something best for healing? Or is it best for patient acceptability? Or is it best because it is the least costly?

Some of these difficulties can be overcome by using clear definitions and by breaking down a question into its constituent parts. However, much of the decision making around this is still subject to good judgement, and questions may need to be refined and updated, depending on likely findings.

Learning activity 3.5 Clinical questions for evidence-based learning and practice

Think about your professional practice.

- Is there an issue you would like to know more about?
- Have your colleagues or patients asked you a question you don't know the answer to, or are unsure about?
- How do you think you could phrase a question to try to find the answer?
- Think about how you define the words you use. Are there different ways of saying the same thing?
- What aspect is the most important? If you want to know if something is better than something else, how are you going to define 'better'?

Write down your question, and check whether it captures all the key elements you need to be able to answer it.

- If it's not quite right, try to refine and rewrite it.
- Then try a search engine you have access to and see how well it works at finding the answer. This could be a general internet search engine or one provided by your employer or academic institution.
- How successful is your search? Can you find results that help to answer your question?
- If the search doesn't prove very fruitful, try again with different combinations of different search terms.

Once a clear question has been broken down and outlined, the next stage is to systematically search for relevant literature/research sources to find a possible answer. When looking for published information, the key sources are now all web based. These may include a search using keywords in a common online search engine, but it is generally considered more appropriate to use one of several internationally available specific healthcare-related databases. Those most commonly used include the Cumulative Index of Nursing and Allied Healthcare Literature (CINAHL) and Medline, which contains information from the US-based National Library of Medicine. These are preferred to more generic database searches, as they include sources of information which have normally been peer reviewed and are from well-recognised and more reputable sources. Hence, information found through them is likely to be of better quality than that found elsewhere. These are also preferable to printed textbooks, which can quickly become out of date.

Once evidence has been located, the next step is to make a judgement about its value, effectively asking 'is it any good?' This is a really important question, as some types of evidence will be stronger than others, and for great nurses to carry out the best practice they need to be assured that their actions are based on the soundest information available. They also need to consider how the evidence fits with the clinical setting, and their particular patient's circumstances.

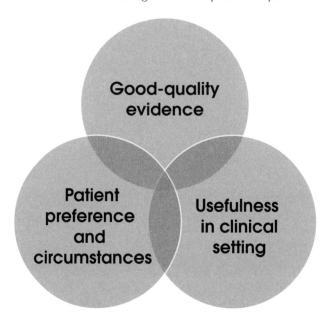

Figure 3.5 Appraisal of evidence sources

There are several detailed ways in which literature-based evidence sources can be appraised. If you would like to know more about this, please have a look at the useful websites listed in Box 3.3 below.

Box 3.3 Useful websites for critical appraisal

Critical Appraisal Skills Programme (2018). https://casp-uk.net/ (last accessed 13.1.2020).

University of York Centre for Reviews and Dissemination (2020). https://www.york.ac.uk/crd/ (last accessed 13.1.2020).

National Institute for Health and Care Excellence (2020). https://www.nice.org.uk/ (last accessed 13.1.2020).

Only when it is clear that the evidence sources located are of the highest quality, and they fit with the needs of the patient and the clinical setting, can the final stage of implementation be taken forward.

Although it is possible for all nurses to carry out comprehensive searches to find different sources of evidence which may answer a particular question (in keeping with the work of

Cochrane), there are now a number of freely available online databases which specialise in summarising key pieces of evidence on many relevant nursing and healthcare topics to make findings easily accessible. These include the Cochrane Library, the Joanna Briggs Institute and the National Institute for Healthcare Excellence (NICE) (see Box 3.4).

Box 3.4 Sources of summaries of evidence/information

http://www.cochranelibrary.com

http://joannabriggs.org/

https://www.nice.org.uk/

Learning activity 3.6

Think about the question you asked in learning activity 3.5 above.

Then have a look at one of the websites in Box 3.3 above and see if you can find an answer there. Don't forget to try various different combinations of different search terms and use the help pages to get help with searching.

Conclusion

Lifelong learning is a major commitment, which all great nurses must undertake and it is essential in order to develop nursing both of the hand and head. It is clear from this overview that lifelong learning can take many forms but it is always crucial in ensuring that the highest standards of nursing care are consistently achieved. In order to be a great nurse, a nurse must deliver great care, and lifelong learning is one of the essential building blocks that supports excellence in nursing practice.

Box 3.5 How to be a great nurse – five steps to lifelong learning

1. Identify your own learning style and use it to help you to learn effectively
2. Take responsibility for your own learning
3. Take every opportunity to learn from others
4. Take every opportunity to learn from yourself and from experience
5. Take every opportunity to learn from evidence

References

Bifarin, O. & Stonehouse, D. (2017). Clinical supervision: an important part of every nurse's practice. *British Journal of Nursing.* **26**(6), 331–35.

Care Quality Commission (CQC) (2013). *Supporting information and guidance: Supporting effective clinical supervision.* https://www.cqc.org.uk/sites/default/files/documents/20130625_800734_v1_00_supporting_information-effective_clinical_supervision_for_publication.pdf (last accessed 13.1.2020).

Cochrane, A. (1972). *Effectiveness and Efficiency. Random reflections on health services. Report on randomised controlled trials (RCTs).* Nuffield Trust.

Crawford, D. & Cannon, E.J. (2018). Peer learning across the curriculum. *Nurse Education Today.* **65**, 239–41.

Dewey, J. (1938). *Experience and education*. New York: Macmillan.

Felstead, I.S. & Springett, K. (2014). An exploration of role model influence on adult nursing students' professional development: a phenomenological research study. *Nurse Education Today.* **37**, 66–70.

Honey, P. & Mumford, A. (1986). *The manual of learning styles.* Peter Honey Associates.

Hughes, S.J. & Quinn R. (2013). *Principles and practice of nurse education.* 6th edn). Cheltenham: Nelson Thornes.

International Council of Nurses (ICN) (2010). *Career planning and development.* https://www.icn.ch/sites/default/files/inline-files/2010_workbook_Career%20planning%20and%20development_eng.pdf (last accessed 22.1.2020).

International Council of Nurses (ICN) (2012). *Closing the gap: from evidence to action.* http://fliphtml5.com/hqgy/mzmz/basic/51-58 (last accessed 13.1.2020).

Irvine, S., Williams, B. & McKenna, L. (2018). Near peer teaching in undergraduate nurse education: an integrative review. *Nurse Education Today.* **70**, 60–68.

Koivu, A., Saarine, P.I. & Hyrkas, K. (2012). Who benefits from clinical supervision and how? The association between clinical supervision and the work related well being of female hospital nurses. *Journal of Clinical Nursing.* **21**, 2567–78.

Kolb, D. (1984). *Experiential learning as the science of learning and development.* Englewood-Cliffs NJ: Prentice-Hall.

Kolb, D.A. (1976). *The learning style inventory: Technical manual.* Boston, MA: McBer & Co.

Learning Styles (2019). https://www.learning-styles-online.com/overview/ (last accessed 13.1.2020).

Miraglia, R. & Asselin, M. (2015). Reflection as an educational strategy in nursing professional development: An integrative review. *Journal for Nurses in Professional Development.* **31**(2), 6–72.

Nelwati, A.K.L. & Chan, C.M. (2018). A systematic review of qualitative studies exploring peer learning experiences of undergraduate nursing students. *Nurse Education Today.* **71**, 185–92.

New Zealand Nurse Educators Preceptorship Subgroup (2010). *Preceptoring for Excellence. National Framework for Nursing Preceptorship programmes.* https://edu.cdhb.health.nz/Hospitals-Services/Health-Professionals/netp/NetP-Programme-Overview/Documents/National%20Preceptorship%20Framework%20%202010.pdf (last accessed 13.1.2020).

Nursing and Midwifery Council (NMC) (2014). *Standards for competence for registered nurses.* https://www.nmc.org.uk/globalassets/sitedocuments/standards/nmc-standards-for-competence-for-registered-nurses.pdf (last accessed 13.1.2020).

Nursing and Midwifery Council (NMC) (2016). *Revalidation/What you need to do.* http://revalidation.nmc.org.uk/what-you-need-to-do/continuing-professional-development.html (last accessed 13.1.2020).

Nursing and Midwifery Council (2018). *The Code.* https://www.nmc.org.uk/globalassets/sitedocuments/nmc-publications/nmc-code.pdf (last accessed 13.1.2020).

Nursing and Midwifery Council (NMC) (2018a). *Future nurse: Part 1. Standards of proficiency for registered nurses.* https://www.nmc.org.uk/globalassets/sitedocuments/education-standards/future-nurse-proficiencies.pdf (last accessed 13.1.2020).

Nursing and Midwifery Council (NMC) (2018b) *Part 2. Standards for student supervision and assessment.* https://www.nmc.org.uk/standards-for-education-and-training/standards-for-student-supervision-and-assessment/ (last accessed 13.1.2020).

Nursing and Midwifery Council (NMC) (2018c) *Part 3. Standards for pre-registration nursing programmes*. https://www.nmc.org.uk/standards/standards-for-nurses/standards-for-pre-registration-nursing-programmes/ (last accessed 13.1.2020).

Royal College of Nursing (RCN) (2017). *Guidance for mentors of nursing and midwifery students*. https://www.rcn.org.uk/professional-development/publications/pub-006133 (last accessed 13.1.2020).

Schön, D.A. (1983). *The reflective practitioner. How professionals think in action*. USA: Basic Books.

Spencer, S. (2009). *The 'curious practitioner': effective lifelong learning. Nursing in Practice*. https://www.nursinginpractice.com/%E2%80%9Ccurious-practitioner%E2%80%9D-effective-lifelong-learning (last accessed 13.1.2020).

The Interprofessional CPD and Lifelong Learning UK Working Group (2019). *Principles for continuing professional development and lifelong learning in health and social care*. https://www.bda.uk.com/training/cpd/cpdjointstatement (last accessed 13.1.2020).

Recommended reading on searching for evidence

Aveyard, H. (2014). *Doing a literature review in health and social care: a practical guide.* Maidenhead: Open University Press.

Aveyard, H., Sharp, P. & Woolliams, M. (2015). *A beginner's guide to critical thinking and writing in health and social care.* 2nd edn. Maidenhead: McGraw Hill.

Cullum, N. (2008). *Evidence-based nursing: an introduction.* Oxford: Wiley Blackwell.

Gerrish, K. & Lacey, M. (2010). *The research process in nursing.* Oxford: Wiley Blackwell.

Le May, A. & Holmes, S. (2012). *Introduction to nursing research: developing research awareness.* London: Hodder Arnold.

Recommended reading on learning from self

Jasper, M. (2013). *Beginning reflective practice.* 2nd edn. Andover: Cengage Learning.

Chapter 4

Effective nursing

Introduction

Looking back at the definition of 'nursing' and 'nurse' in Chapter 1 (pp. 1,2), it is evident that the role of the nurse is complex and influenced by many factors. Great nursing involves being effective. Being effective as a nurse means being able to provide skilful nursing care that gives the best chance of achieving the desired results for the patient and their family. It is important to acknowledge that measuring effectiveness is more complex than simply focusing on what the nurse does and the results of that action; effectiveness may mean different things to the nurse, the patient, the patient's family and other members of the team. Great nurses can be effective in many different contexts.

Being skilful means being able to respond flexibly to changing circumstances, with the aim of successfully achieving the goals of nursing care (Kagan *et al.* 1986). This requires a high level of competence and effectiveness in the nursing tasks, or interventions, so that performing them has a positive impact on the health and wellbeing of those in the nurse's care. Competence in carrying out nursing skills is based on sound knowledge, good communication, emotional intelligence and appropriate attitudes, as well as the 'head, heart and hand' approach discussed already. The acquisition of knowledge through lifelong learning was considered in Chapter 3, and this chapter explores some of the fundamental ingredients that make up the skills, of good (effective) nursing.

Developing, enhancing and updating practical skills

Nursing is a profession. The meanings of the terms 'professional' and 'professionalism' suggest that an individual who belongs to a given profession possesses the values, skills and competency required for that particular field. To be a great nurse involves having, developing and maintaining an effective set of skills that enable the nurse to meet the needs of patients. As discussed briefly in Chapter 1, effective nursing involves the use of practical skills that achieve positive health outcomes for the patient, underpinned by the core values discussed in Chapter 2, and the commitment to lifelong learning outlined in Chapter 3. These skills are gradually developed over time, by gaining knowledge and understanding of the theory underpinning the skill, undertaking the skill as a learner and gradually incorporating that skill into daily practice while increasing the degree of effectiveness and competence/proficiency with which the skill is carried out.

Many definitions of the term 'skill' describe it as a work activity that requires specific training, knowledge and experience. It is also synonymous with the ability to do something well. However, the skills required of effective nurses are immense and diverse. A glance at the standards for proficiency of registered nurses in the UK (NMC 2019) demonstrates this complex spectrum of skills, and a closer look at these standards reveals some of the generic skills that are expected of nurses on registration, focusing on a nurse's role as a practitioner, educator, leader and researcher (see Learning activity 4.1).

Learning activity 4.1 Future nurse: Standards for proficiency of registered nurses

Consider the following extract from the NMC (2019, p.3) Standards for proficiency of registered nurses:

> 'Registered nurses play a vital role in providing, leading and coordinating care that is compassionate, evidence-based, and person-centred. They are accountable for their own actions and must be able to work autonomously, or as an equal partner, with a range of other professionals, and in interdisciplinary teams. In order to respond to the impact and demands of professional nursing practice, they must be emotionally intelligent and resilient individuals, who are able to manage their own personal health and wellbeing and know when and how to access support.
>
> Registered nurses make an important contribution to the promotion of health, health protection and the prevention of ill health. They do this by empowering people, communities and populations to exercise choice, take control of their own health decisions and behaviours, and by supporting people to manage their own care where possible.
>
> Registered nurses provide leadership in the delivery of care for people of all ages and from different backgrounds, cultures and beliefs. They provide nursing care for people who have complex mental, physical, cognitive and behavioural care needs, those living with dementia, the elderly, and for people at the end of their life. They must be able to care for people in their own home, in the community or hospital or in any healthcare settings where their needs are supported and managed. They work in the context of continual change, challenging environments, different models of care delivery, shifting demographics, innovation, and rapidly evolving technologies. Increasing integration of health and social care services will require registered nurses to negotiate boundaries and play a proactive role in interdisciplinary teams. The confidence and ability to think critically, apply knowledge and skills, and provide expert, evidence-based, direct nursing care therefore lies at the centre of all registered nursing practice.'

- Identify five to ten skills (there may well be more), at any level, that you can see being suggested as central to effective nursing here.
- Assess your own need for further development of such skills and make a plan for doing so. Be honest with yourself about areas in which you could improve.

On graduation/registration, nurses are expected to have a full set of fundamental clinical skills and to be proficient in these skills. In the UK, the NMC (2019) operationalise these through seven platforms listed in Box 4.1. This is a summary of the skills which are considered essential to all fields of nursing and fundamental to effective practice, with similar proficiencies identified by other professional regulatory bodies globally. Guidance for developing and performing a skill for different fields and specialties within nursing can be found in multiple texts and other sources.

Box 4.1 Seven platforms of proficiency for registered nurses (NMC 2019)

1. Being an accountable professional
2. Promoting health and preventing ill-health
3. Assessing needs and planning care
4. Providing and evaluating care
5. Leading and managing nursing care and working in teams
6. Improving safety and quality of care
7. Coordinating care.

Further information and details of the outcome statements for each platform have been designed to apply across all four UK fields of nursing practice (adult, children, learning disabilities, mental health) and all care settings and can be viewed at:
https://www.nmc.org.uk/globalassets/sitedocuments/education-standards/future-nurse-proficiencies.pdf

Nursing is an 'applied' discipline, using knowledge gained from sociology, psychology, biology, pathology and other branches of sciences, and applying it to the reality of clinical practice and to the 'head, heart and hand' approach. It is often said that the most effective nurses are 'knowledgeable doers' who are capable of competent practice, based on an awareness of theory and evidence, using a combination of 'knowing that' (theoretical knowledge) and 'knowing how' (practical knowledge) (Benner 1984), combined with practical experience that enables them to continuously develop and improve their skills throughout their career. The development of nursing education has been largely driven by this 'knowledgeable doer' approach to practitioner skill development.

The development of skills in nursing is usually described using Benner's (1984) application to nursing of Dreyfus' model of skills acquisition based on a continuum of personal development from 'novice to expert'. This has been the basis for the development of nursing education over the last few decades (as briefly discussed in Chapter 2). According to this approach, the development of any skill passes through five levels of proficiency (see Figure 4.1 at the end of this section): novice; advanced beginner, competent, proficient and expert. These five levels can vary, depending on the skill involved and the stage of the nurse's education or career. Student nurses, for example, may move from novice to advanced beginner by the end of their first placement in many fundamental skills, but they may still be novices in more complex or advanced activities. On arrival at the next placement, they may need to return to novice status when they encounter new skills not previously learned. A newly qualified nurse may have reached competence in many skills, but will need to develop new skills once they settle into their first post-qualifying post, as expectations of them will have changed. They may therefore return to advanced beginner or even novice in some aspects of their role as they continue to develop their effectiveness.

Novice nurses

Novice nurses have no experience of providing nursing care, although some may enter the nursing profession with experience of caring in other formal and informal roles. A novice needs to develop the fundamental skills of nursing and caring in order to be fully effective. These fundamental skills are focused on providing essential aspects of care such as communication, assessment, observation and monitoring, hygiene care, supporting activities of daily living, preventing infection. Novice nurses are taught how to carry out these tasks and are given opportunities to practise them in highly supervised situations until they are deemed able to carry out the tasks safely and effectively without supervision. The performance of these activities is underpinned by a fundamental knowledge of common situations in which they are needed, based on a prescribed set of rules and with only limited contextual understanding. Novice nurses are not expected to act with their own initiative; they are simply expected to follow the guidance given by those supervising them.

Advanced beginners

Advanced beginners have successfully practised a skill sufficiently for them to be able to carry it out safely and with minimal supervision. Their performance is deemed to be acceptable. The situations in which the practice takes place are still new and the nurse must still think about the rules governing the task, but their experience of carrying out the activity is increasing, as is their confidence and effectiveness. Support and feedback are still needed from a more experienced practitioner who is, at least, competent in the activity. The nurse will need to practise the skill much more so that they can do it well without having to think about the rules. They will struggle to perform the skill in situations that are different from the ones they have already experienced frequently. For example, at this stage the nurse will be much more confident in their ability to communicate with patients effectively and, equally, the patient will be more confident in them.

Competent practitioners

Competent practitioners have often developed their competence in specific skills and tasks over several years. The skill is performed consistently and effectively under various circumstances and with reasonable planning, but without the communication, speed, confidence, mastery and flexibility that would be demonstrated by a proficient nurse.

Proficient nurses

Proficient nurses can carry out a skill or task with a deep understanding and appreciation of the whole context surrounding the skill and its execution. They understand the long-term goals of the interaction and its likely impact on outcomes for patients. The proficient nurse has learnt from experience what to expect, and can adapt the way they act and communicate, according to the responses of patients and others. They can also practise the skill in situations that are not in keeping with expected situations or results.

Expert nurses

Expert nurses have had many years' experience of undertaking a skill and have continued to develop their mastery of it over time. They have an intuitive appreciation of the situations in which the skill is carried out and they no longer rely on rules or guidelines but are able to adapt their activity and communication style according to situations as they present themselves. Intuition is often involved in the decisions made relating to the skill.

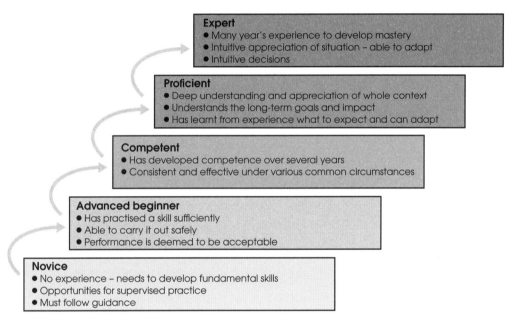

Figure 4.1 The Dreyfus model of skills acquisition applied to nursing (Benner 1984)

Learning activity 4.2 From competent to expert

Write about a skill that you have seen performed by another nurse at the level of 'competence', as described by Benner (see above).

● What did you see the nurse do, under what circumstances and with what results?

● How effective was it?

● What was the context?

● Why do you feel that the 'competence' level was demonstrated?

Now think about how the nurse would need to be able to demonstrate the same skill at the level of:

a. Proficient

b. Expert.

Now think about yourself and a skill that at one time, you were a novice in.

- Where are you in terms of the level now? Advanced beginner? Competent? Proficient? Expert?
- What would you need to be able to do in order to demonstrate effectiveness in that skill at the next level up?

In 2019 the Nursing and Midwifery Council in the UK chose to use the term 'proficiency', rather than 'competency', in its new *Standards of proficiency of registered nurses* (NMC 2019) to reflect the terminology in Benner's model. These proficiencies reflect what newly registered nurses are expected to know and be capable of doing in order to be considered safe and competent but not necessarily expert.

Nursing care quality

Effectiveness in healthcare is linked with quality. Having the correct nursing skills does not necessarily mean that the quality of care provided is excellent, or even that it is effective, as there are many factors that contribute to excellent care. Some of these factors are beyond the control of the individual nurse (despite how great that individual's practice is) and may involve other influences such as care systems, the way nurses are educated and how care is led, managed and funded. Aiken *et al.* (2014), for example, have demonstrated that patient outcomes following surgery are positively influenced by the level of education of nurses, their skills and staffing levels.

Great nurses are central to quality healthcare because of the significant influence they have on the patient experience through the 'head, heart and hand' approach. Without effective nursing, the goals of excellent healthcare cannot be met. Unfortunately, most media stories about nursing care are negative, giving the impression that nursing is a profession with declining standards (Watson 2012). This is not necessarily because nursing care is poor or ineffective – often, on the contrary – but news stories tend not to focus on the positive aspects because of society's interest in negativity and the fact that media stories are of greater interest to the public if they are shocking or sensational. Most nurses provide excellent and effective care nearly all the time. It is important, therefore, that they can demonstrate how effective their care is, and the difference it makes to patients, by developing their own approach to assuring quality in what they do.

High-quality, or excellent, care is the right of everyone and falls into six main domains (Everett & Wright 2015). These reflect some of the nursing values discussed in Chapters 1 and 2:

- Person-(patient-)centred: focused on the individual receiving care and their family
- Safe: does not do harm
- Effective: achieves the aims and goals of care
- Efficient: well-organised, competent and avoiding waste
- Equitable: meeting everyone's needs in a fair and just way, respecting the uniqueness of each person
- Timely: proving care when it is needed and without delay.

There are two main views of nursing care quality:
1. The perceptions of the givers of care, the nurses, themselves
2. The experiences and perceptions of those receiving care, the patients.

From both these views, it is important that there is objective evidence of quality of care and that any deficits are acted upon to improve it. There have been many systems and processes in place that aim to measure the quality of patient care. Recently, for example, monitoring and improving care quality in the National Health Service (NHS) in England has been the responsibility of NHS Improvement (https://improvement.nhs.uk/). Because nurses provide so much care within the NHS, the nursing contribution to quality is often the focus. Although nurses work as part of a wider multidisciplinary team, it is important that they are also able to articulate the impact nursing care has on patient outcomes and that standards of nursing care are specifically measured. The processes of measuring and monitoring nursing care, with a view to maintaining standards of care or making improvements, are often referred to as 'Nursing Metrics', 'Nursing Quality Indicators', or 'Patient outcome measures' (McSherry, McSherry & Watson 2012).

Measurable care quality indicators, with a specific focus on the quality and impact of nursing care, are often referred to as 'nursing metrics.' Maben *et al.* (2012) found that the most commonly cited nursing care quality indicators currently focus on five areas:

- Healthcare-associated infections
- Pressure ulcers
- Falls
- Drug administration errors
- Patient complaints.

They focus on these areas because they are relatively easy to measure, but such indicators are unlikely to reflect the true complexity of nursing and its influence on patient care quality, as they are mainly concerned with 'hand and head' rather than 'heart'. Another problem with these indicators is their overt focus on acute adult nursing care and not on, for example, care quality in mental health, community or children's nursing. Hence, much work is needed to develop indicators that reflect the breadth of the nursing role and its complexity as well as its influence on patient outcomes. Care quality indicators for nursing need to be developed in a coordinated way so that different nursing teams' results can be compared to those of others (locally, nationally and internationally). This will enable benchmarking to take place so that the full range of nursing activities (across hand, head and heart) are examined. The information gathered through such processes also needs to be transparent so that those receiving care know what to expect.

Interpersonal skills and nurse–patient relationships

Interpersonal skills are those aspects of communication and social skills that are needed when developing relationships in direct person-to-person contact with others and they are key to the 'heart' of much nursing practice. It is through interpersonal processes (closely linked with the idea of emotional intelligence discussed in Chapter 2) that nurses are able to develop effective 'therapeutic relationships' with those for whom they provide care. These interpersonal skills are used to build the respect, rapport and trust (Allender & Spradley 2005) that is needed to enable nurses to work effectively with patients and other team members.

In an integrative review of the literature, Kornhaber *et al.* (2016, p. 537) defined a therapeutic interpersonal relationship as 'One which is perceived by patients to encompass caring, and supportive non-judgmental behaviour, embedded in a safe environment during an often stressful period' and described these important relationships as:

1. Lasting for a brief moment in time or continuing for extended periods
2. Involving a display of warmth, friendliness, genuine interest, empathy, and the wish to facilitate and support
3. Engendering a climate for interactions that facilitate effective communication
4. Associated with improvements in patient satisfaction, adherence to treatment, quality of life, levels of anxiety and depression, and decreased healthcare cost.

Conversely, negative clinician–patient relationships are associated with increased psychological distress and feelings of dehumanisation.

Communication and interpersonal skills

Effective, high-quality nursing care that facilitates the development of therapeutic interpersonal relationships is significantly associated with the way nurses communicate and interact with those in their care. Communication is a fundamental aspect of interpersonal 'heart' skills and helps nurses to demonstrate compassion, empathy, respect and trust and develop rapport with patients, families and other health professionals. Many patient complaints about nursing care are focused on communication problems and how these reflect poor attitudes and a lack of fundamental nursing values. Great nurses embody Egan's (1982) description of someone who is a 'skilled helper'. Anyone can help another person, but some are formally given the challenging role of helping others deal with life's problems and crises.

In 'helping' professions such as nursing and other health and social care roles, it is not sufficient simply to have technical skills that enable the practitioner to undertake specific helping tasks. Additional skills are needed to provide holistic care and help individuals overcome emotional and psychological challenges. For example, it may seem relatively simple to help an older person to wash and dress (Hand), but to carry out such an intervention in a way that understands their needs (Head), respects their dignity and uses the situation to engage with the patient on a personal level (Heart), so that a respectful, trusting relationship is built, is much more complex. Every situation faced by nurses requires the ability to develop relationships with patients involving the use of exceptional communication skills. Alongside compassion and professionalism, it has often been argued that without exceptionally effective communication and relationship building, good nursing is impossible (Hogg & Hanley 2018).

Communication is a fundamental part of life. It happens in millions of different ways in both the human and animal world. It is how we ask questions, understand others and make judgements and decisions. It is the process that enables the world to be harmonious, and without it, life is chaotic. It therefore stands to reason that good communication is an essential component of effective nursing.

It is the process through which nurses can understand the needs of patients and their families, give information and provide advice. Patients can inform nurses and other members of the team how they feel, what they need, what is working and what is not, and nurses can, if they listen carefully, act according to this information. Communication is the basis of the 'therapeutic relationship' between the nurse and the patient, which aims to identify and meet patients' health needs and to improve their health and wellbeing (Candlin 2008). Without it, the goals of nursing cannot be achieved, and care will be ineffective, placing patients at risk of harm. Being able to communicate in a manner which best serves patient needs is an essential nursing skill; and lack of effective communication is the most common reason for nurses' failure to provide care that meets patients' needs. In all fields of nursing, communication and relationship management skills are an integral part of global nursing competencies; and in the UK, the NMC (2019) *Standards of proficiency for registered nurses* highlight the importance of communication in providing safe, compassionate, person-centred care.

Great nurses often act as a 'hub', bringing together the communication process that surrounds every patient and which may include many different senders and receivers of messages, including the patient, their family, other health professionals, and social care agency workers. The most common model used to explain the process of communication in nursing is that developed by Shannon and Weaver (1949) who presented communication as a two-way process of 'sending', 'encoding' (turning thoughts and ideas into communication), 'receiving' and 'responding' to messages (see Figure 4.2). This linear model, suggesting that each stage happens one after the other, makes the process of communication sound relatively simple, even though, in healthcare situations, communication is complicated by the need for many messages to be sent and received at once. Such a model, however, helps nurses to understand how communication happens and what can go wrong.

Communication is initiated by a 'sender' who can be a healthcare professional, patient, family member, or any other person involved in their care. Having 'encoded' the message (constructed it in a way that is likely to be understandable to the receiver), the sender conveys a message which has meaning both to the sender and the 'receiver'. The message represents information, ideas, instructions and so on. Such messages are often conveyed using symbols such as language or pictures representing the meaning of the message. The means by which the sender conveys the message is referred to as the 'channel' (see Table 4.1); this is the mode of communication, which can be verbal, non-verbal or written.

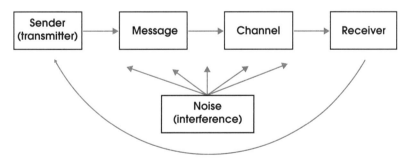

Figure 4.2 Linear process model of communication (Shannon & Weaver 1949)

Communication is facilitated through several different methods (see Table 4.1) that are often used in combination, particularly in the case of verbal and non-verbal; often the words someone is saying convey a different message to that of the facial expression of the message sender. It is well known that the communication of verbal information can easily be forgotten or remembered incorrectly, so verbal messages can also be provided in written form to support memory of such verbal information and, increasingly, written information is sent electronically. The process of communication is not one-way, and the 'receiver' provides feedback to the sender, making them interchangeable within the process. All stages of the process are affected by interference ('noise'), or barriers, which affect the clarity and understanding of the message. Recognising and overcoming communication barriers is essential in providing effective care to people who have difficulty communicating. Barriers can arise in any part of the communication process and vary depending on the method of communication (see Table 4.1).

Table 4.1 Channels/methods of communication

Method of communication	Meaning and use	Examples of potential barriers/problems
Verbal	Using the spoken language to convey messages, including the tone and volume of voice. This frequently and increasingly can mean verbal communication using telephones, computers and other methods of non-face-to-face communication. This is often seen as the most obvious form of communication but may be affected by many factors.	• Hearing difficulties • Speech and language problems • Cultural differences • Environmental distractions such as noise • Internal distractions such as stress • Memory and cognitive problems
Non-verbal	Employing facial expression, eye contact or touch as a means of expressing thoughts feelings and attitudes. Non-verbal messages are usually provided at the same time as verbal information, but non-verbal messages can also work in isolation. A smile, or sympathetic expression, for example, can have a positive impact, in the same way as a frown or aggressive expression can have the opposite effect. Non-verbal expression can convey different messages from those given verbally at the same time, and this may confuse the receiver. Misinterpretation of non-verbal messages is common. Active listening is an important part of non-verbal communication.	• Sight problems • Cultural differences • Attitudes of the sender
Written	This includes the use of written electronic forms of communication such as email and social media.	• Reading ability • Ability to receive and store messages • Clarity of the message

Communication in different situations

Different styles, and complexity, of communication are often used by skilled nurses in different situations, depending on the needs of the patient and the clinical situation. Effective communication is always an essential aspect of great nursing practice, but there are some circumstances in which the nurse needs to pay special attention to *how* they communicate, particularly when the situation is complex. Some examples follow (see Trenoweth & Allymamod (2015) for others).

1. First contact: A relatively simple process of asking questions may be used to find out about the history and symptoms when a patient presents for assessment following a minor injury. Having made introductions, the nurse will ask both closed and open questions, to elicit what has happened to the patient and what the effect has been so that an assessment of the nature and extent of the injury can be made and a plan for diagnosis and treatment can be put in place. Meeting a patient or client for the first time is an important opportunity to ensure that they get a positive first impression of the setting and professionals working there. If the first impression is not managed carefully, the person may find it difficult to trust those caring for them in the future. Greeting the patient in a friendly, professional manner is essential. This is particularly important when working with children, for their future confidence in healthcare.

2. High stress situations: Recognising that receiving healthcare is a stressful event for most people is an important part of the care process. Examples of such situations include: admission to hospital or for an unpleasant procedure or investigation, undergoing surgery, and having a health assessment for the first time. In such circumstances, communicating effectively can help to reduce stress significantly. This should involve giving simple, clear explanations about what will happen.

3. Giving bad news: Being informed of bad news is highly distressing, and in some settings it is very likely that the nurse will have to break this news to the patient. A more complex approach to communication is needed if the nurse is working with a patient who has recently, for example, been given the news that they have a chronic health condition which will require long-term care and treatment. This will be bad news for the patient, and they will need careful explanations and checking of their understanding.

4. Patients with cognitive problems: Being unable to concentrate on what is being said, or remember what has been said, can make the care process very stressful for many patients, as their understanding of the situation is detrimentally affected. People with dementia, learning difficulties, mental health problems and others who find the process of thinking and remembering difficult, need enhanced skills in communication or help from those who have such skills. For instance, patients with cognitive or memory problems, such as those with a learning difficulty or dementia, will require a different approach to communication in the two examples given above (high stress situations and giving bad news). The nurse will need to adapt their communication style and approach to meet the needs of the patient who may not immediately understand what they say and/or may not be able to remember the information later. This may often require a change in the style of verbal language and non-verbal communication cues used and/or the support of a carer or family member.

People use many of these types of communication in their everyday lives concurrently, without necessarily giving them much thought. However, the nature of nursing, and the vulnerability of those receiving care, means that good communication must be used deliberately and with care and thought and in a way that achieves its purposes at all times. Those applying to enter the nursing profession usually have their ability to communicate successfully assessed at interview. However, communication skills are often developed and honed through practice, education and experience over an entire nursing career, and it is important to get this right.

Non-verbal communication

Verbal messages conveyed to patients by nurses can be in opposition to non-verbal communication if the nurse is not skilled in making sure the two match up. A good example of this is asking: 'How are you today?' if this is done in a way that indicates that the nurse is genuinely interested and ready to receive an answer, the patient will feel able to offer information about how they really feel and the nurse will gain valuable information. However, if the messages are mixed and the nurse is not making direct eye contact with the patient or appears to be distracted, the patient is most likely to answer 'I'm fine thanks' when, in fact, they are not. Actively listening to the answers given to an appropriately framed question is vital, and involves good non-verbal communication.

Box 4.2 Two acronyms to assist in learning good non-verbal communication practice

SOLER acronym (Egan 1982)	SURETY acronym (Stickley 2011)
S Sit squarely – face the patient and adopt a posture that indicates interest and involvement	**S Sit at an angle to the person** – indicating an interest in the person and interaction, but without being confrontational
O Open posture – adopt a non-defensive posture that indicates readiness to engage and listen	**U Uncross legs and arms** – indicating openness rather than defensiveness in the communication exchange
L Lean towards the other – indicating engagement and interest in the person	**R Relax** – indicating being comfortable in the interaction
E Eye contact – giving the message that you are fully involved in the interaction but not staring so that the interaction feels threatening	**E Eye contact** – indicating communication, respect and paying attention
R Relax – giving the message that you have time to listen, that it is your priority and that you are confident in what you are doing	**T Touch** – appropriately, to indicate compassion, empathy and understanding
	Y Your intuition

Two examples of non-verbal communication acronyms are provided in Box 4.2 above. Acronyms can help nurses remember the fundamentals of a skill while they learn to integrate it into practice. Stickley (2011) argued that Egan's (1982) SOLER model needed updating and that the use of the SURETY approach (Box 4.2) better facilitated cultural sensitivity and touch in non-verbal communication.

Learning activity 4.3 Applying SOLER and SURETY

Considering these two acronyms for good non-verbal communication, answer the following questions:

- What are the differences between the two?
- What do these differences say about good non-verbal communication in today's healthcare environment?
- Can you see any problems with any of the advice?

Thinking about a recent interaction you had with someone during your working day:

- In what way did that interaction reflect, or not, either (or both) of these two approaches?

Communicating with other team members

An essential aspect of communication in healthcare is that which takes place between health professionals – that is, between members of the wider interdisciplinary team as well as the nursing team. This communication is an essential aspect of effective patient care and safety as it is the means by which patient information is transferred between different team members. Nurses are often the co-ordinators of information since they tend to be the team members who have the most direct patient contact.

Within the nursing team itself, the two most important methods of communication are:

- Care documentation, reflecting the nursing process (assessment, planning, implementation and evaluation – APIE)
- Nursing handovers (sometimes known as 'hand offs') between different nurses and shift teams.

If either of these processes are inadequate, there is a risk of failures in care because of lack of accurate information about the patient. Poor communication is a common cause of patient safety incidents as well as complaints.

Situation, Background, Assessment, Recommendations (SBAR) is a widely used tool for structured communication between health professionals about a patient's condition. This was adapted from the system used in aviation and military settings and is designed to ensure that information is shared in an accurate, precise and effective way. This approach has been used successfully in many critical and emergency healthcare situations as well as in general day-to-day care situations. It is now seen as a useful standardised approach to communicating between individuals in healthcare teams to enable safe and effective transfer of information between individual team members (Müller *et al.* 2018). See Learning activity 4.4 for further information.

Learning activity 4.4 The SBAR tool for health professional communication

NHS improvement in the UK provides an overview of the SBAR (Situation, Background, Assessment, Recommendations) tool at the following link: https://improvement.nhs.uk/resources/sbar-communication-tool/

On p. 7 of this document, some examples of situations in which SBAR can be useful are provided.

Thinking about your recent experience of practice, write your own example of when SBAR was useful, or would have been useful (if you did not use it at the time).

Consider the following questions:

● How does SBAR protect patient safety?

● What might still go wrong, even if SBAR is used?

● What specific skills are needed to be effective when using SBAR?

● How can SBAR save time for nurses?

● How can SBAR support patient advocacy?

In what way did that interaction reflect, or not, either (or both) of these two approaches?

Communication within the multidisciplinary team is an essential component of effective care delivery as it ensures that the team members are all working towards the same goal. In the UK this is highlighted in section 8 of the NMC *Code* (2015) – see Box 4.3.

Box 4.3 *The Code* (NMC 2015) Section 8: Work co-operatively

To achieve this, you must:

8.1 respect the skills, expertise and contributions of your colleagues, referring matters to them when appropriate

8.2 maintain effective communication with colleagues

8.3 keep colleagues informed when you are sharing the care of individuals with other health and care professionals and staff

8.4 work with colleagues to evaluate the quality of your work and that of the team

8.5 work with colleagues to preserve the safety of those receiving care

8.6 share information to identify and reduce risk

8.7 be supportive of colleagues who are encountering health or performance problems. However, this support must never compromise or be at the expense of patient or public safety

In the complex world of healthcare, nurses often act as the coordinator of the patient's care, serving as the link between members of the healthcare team and acting in a liaison role. This is a complex role that cannot be successfully performed without effective communication within the team as well as an understanding of the role of other team members and respect for their contribution. Included in the team is the patient's family and other non-professional carers, who have an even more important contribution to make that is often not acknowledged (partnership working is considered in more detail in Chapter 7). While effective team communication can have a positive impact on patient outcomes, ineffective communication within the team has often been shown to lead to patient harm and dissatisfaction.

Nurses are often not only the coordinators of the multidisciplinary team but can also have a significant influence on team effectiveness. O'Daniel and Rosenstein (2008) proposed that the components of effective teamwork, leading to patient-centred care, included:

- Open communication
- Non-punitive environment
- Clear direction
- Clear and known roles and tasks for team members
- Respectful atmosphere
- Shared responsibility for team success
- Appropriate balance of member participation for the task at hand
- Acknowledgment and processing of conflict
- Clear specifications regarding authority and accountability
- Clear and known decision-making procedures
- Regular and routine communication and information sharing
- Enabling environment, including access to needed resources
- Mechanism to evaluate outcomes and adjust accordingly.

Each item on this list involves effective communication. Many of the general principles of good communication with patients and families discussed earlier also apply to effective interprofessional relationships and embody effective use of the 'head, heart and hand' approach to great nursing.

Using evidence for effective practice

In Chapter 3, we considered the use of evidence as one element which supports the great nurse to undertake lifelong learning. In this chapter, the focus is on the role of evidence as one of the core elements underpinning effective practice. It is essential that evidence gained from research forms a part of the communication and decision-making cycle that makes practice effective and supports the development of therapeutic relationships, and that this evidence is used to enhance both interprofessional and multidisciplinary working.

The use of research evidence to inform practice clearly needs to be balanced with the practice skills, expertise and experience of the nurse, the interpersonal skills used by the nurse to build a meaningful relationship with the patient, the needs of the individual, and their specific circumstances and environment. However, emphasis on the use of 'evidence-based practice' has resulted in some misconceptions about the relative values of these elements in producing effective practice and has, in some cases, led to reduced emphasis on the more heart-orientated nursing skills such as intuition, communication and the skills used when developing positive therapeutic relationships.

The need to base nursing practice on the best available evidence is enshrined within the professional standards of all registered nurses across the globe (ICN 2012). As a means of establishing new knowledge, and moving away from practice based on ritual, routine and personal subjective preference, evidence can clearly support positive changes in patient care, along with improved patient outcomes. However, the use of research evidence needs to be thought through carefully and balanced with other key elements that are essential to providing effective nursing care.

Focusing solely on the use of research evidence as the main factor impacting on a nurse's decision- making when caring for patients has led to many criticisms. One major criticism has arisen from the development of a hierarchy of evidence, which places certain types of research at the pinnacle of knowledge, reduces the nurse's expertise to the lowest level, and completely excludes issues involving communication, relationship building and any input from partnership working with patients and their carers. This hierarchy is commonly illustrated in the following way (see Figure 4.3).

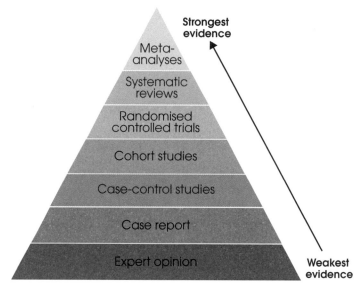

Figure 4.3 The hierarchy of evidence

Placing highly complex research methods (such as meta-analysis, systematic reviews and randomised controlled trials) at the highest levels of this evidence hierarchy ensures that 'evidence' is almost automatically restricted to those subjects and topics which are amenable to being investigated using those methods. Given the diverse nature of nursing and people who need nursing care, this emphasis excludes many areas of practice and patient need, as well as other less sophisticated forms of research investigation. This emphasis also leads to many potential sources of bias, including the financial cost of complex research studies, which ensures that funding is normally provided by those with a vested interest in the area being investigated. This helps to explain the remote and highly controlled nature of these types of studies (with findings that are not directly transferable to real-world situations) and the cultural predominance of studies which take place using healthy male volunteers from first world countries (Sheridan & Julian 2016).

When focusing on the role of evidence-based care in relation to effective nursing practice, individual needs, communication skills, and therapeutic nursing, there have also been a number of very specific criticisms (Baumann 2010):

1. Evidence-based practice does not fit well with individualised holistic patient care
2. Evidence-based practice does not fit well with patient empowerment
3. Evidence-based practice can lead to the development of rigid protocols
4. The scope of evidence-based practice is limited to more medicalised elements of care
5. The place of nursing experience and expertise is marginalised.

In order to be an effective nurse, it is clear that evidence has a role, just as evidence is one element of a nurse's path to lifelong learning. However, to be a great and effective nurse, it is also essential to be aware of the limitations of evidence-based practice, to avoid an over -emphasis on its value, and to place findings from evidence-based research studies within a wider context. Effective nurses can be anywhere on the continuum from novice to expert and they can communicate with their patients in many ways, but the key to developing and maintaining effective therapeutic relationships with patients is to use evidence as only one element in what makes up effective nursing care. As DiCenso, *et al.* (1998, p. 40) argue:

> 'the ultimate goal of nursing is to deliver to patients the best available care … the application of research findings to practice goes hand in hand with clinical expertise and with patient preferences and values.'

The relative worth of all these elements – experience, expertise, communication skills, relationship building, resources and evidence – needs to be balanced for each individual patient in each specific situation. Great, effective nursing care is achieved when this balance is met, achieving that complex mix of 'head, hand and heart' that ensures the patient receives the best available care, tailored to their personal needs, based on the nurse's experience, skills and knowledge of what constitutes best practice and clear communication channels between the patient, their carers and all members of the multidisciplinary team.

Conclusion

Effective practice in nursing is based on an understanding of the importance of expertise, effective communication and the balanced use of evidence. Great nurses are recognised as members of a profession because they have a set of skills which they employ in delivering effective care that impacts positively on patients' health and wellbeing. Effectiveness and competence in such skills are developed over time, through education and experience. Central to the breadth and reach of these skills is the ability of great nurses to develop effective therapeutic interpersonal relationships through excellent communication. Such communication includes that which is needed to be effective in multidisciplinary team working.

The key points in this chapter can best be summarised in six characteristics that are essential for all great nurses – see Box 4.4

Box 4.4 How to be a great nurse: effective nursing

1. Effective nurses are aware of their own areas of expertise and how to use them in many complex situations.

2. Excellence in nursing is achieved by those who constantly develop and improve their skills.

3. Great nurses understand that excellent communication skills are key to effective practice.

4. Effective nurses can adapt their communication skills to a range of challenging situations.

5. Great nurses work effectively in a team.

6. Effective nurses make critical balanced use of research evidence to support best individualised patient care.

Recommendations for further study

Candlin, S. (2008). *Therapeutic Communication: A lifespan approach*. Pearson Australia.

Maben, J., Morrow, E., Ball, J., Robert G. & Griffiths, P. (2012). *High Quality Care Metrics for Nursing*. National Nursing Research Unit, King's College London. https://www.kcl.ac.uk/nmpc/research/nnru/publications/Reports/High-Quality-Care-Metrics-for-Nursing----Nov-2012.pdf (27.1.2020).

Trenoweth, S. & Allymamod, W. (2015). 'Communication and interpersonal skills in challenging circumstances' in: Delves-Yates, C. (ed.) *Essentials of Nursing Practice*. pp. 223–38. London: Sage.

References

Aiken, L., Sloane, D., Bruyneel, L., Van den Heede, K., Griffiths, P., Busse, R., Diomidous, M., Kinnunen, J., Kózka, M., Lesaffre, E., McHugh, M., Moreno-Casbas, M., Rafferty, A., Schwendimann, R., Scott, P., Tishelman, C., van Achterberg, T. & Sermeus, W. (2014). Nurse staffing and education and hospital mortality in nine European countries: a retrospective observational study. *Lancet*. **383**(9931), 1824–30.

Allender, J.S. & Spradley, W. (2005). *Community health nursing: Promoting and protecting the public's health*. 6th edn. Philadelphia: Lippincott.

Baumann, S.L. (2010). The limitations of evidence based practice. *Nursing Science Quarterly*. **23**(3), 226–30.

Benner, P. (1984). *From Novice to Expert. Excellence and power in clinical nursing practice*. Menlo Park, CA: Addison-Wesley.

Candlin, S. (2008). *Therapeutic communication: A lifespan approach*. New South Wales: Pearson Australia.

DiCenso, A., Cullum, N. & Ciliska, D. (1998). Implementing evidence based nursing: some misconceptions. *Evidence Based Nursing*. **1**(2), 38–40

Egan, G. (1982). *The skilled helper*. 2nd edn. Monterey, CA: Brooks/Cole.

Everett, F. & Wright, W. (2015). 'Delivering effective care' in Delves-Yates, C. (ed.) *Essentials of nursing practice*. pp. 143–156. London: Sage.

Hogg, R. & Hanley, J. (2018). Learning lessons from the analysis of patient complaints relating to staff attitudes, behaviour and communication, using the concept of emotional labour. *Journal of Clinical Nursing.* **27**(5–6) e1004–12 https://doi.org/10.1111/jocn.14121 (last accessed 16.1.2020).

International Council of Nurses (ICN) (2012). *Closing the gap: from evidence to action.* http://fliphtml5.com/hqgy/mzmz/basic/51-58 (last accessed 16.1.2020).

Kagan, C., Evans, J. & Kay, B. (1986). *A manual of interpersonal skills for nurses.* London: Harper and Row.

Kornhaber, R., Walsh, K., Duff, J. & Walker, K. (2016). Enhancing adult therapeutic interpersonal relationships in the acute care setting: an integrative review. *Journal of Multidisciplinary Healthcare.* **9**: 53 –46 doi:10.2147/JMDH.S116957

Maben, J., Morrow, E., Ball, J., Robert, G. & Griffiths, P. (2012). *High Quality Care Metrics for Nursing.* National Nursing Research Unit, King's College London. https://www.kcl.ac.uk/nmpc/research/nnru/publications/Reports/High-Quality-Care-Metrics-for-Nursing----Nov-2012.pdf (last accessed 16.1.2020).

McSherry, W., McSherry, R. & Watson, R. (eds) (2012). *Care in nursing. Principles, values and skills.* Oxford: Oxford University Press.

Müller, M., Jürgens, J., Redaèlli, M., *et al.* (2018). Impact of the communication and patient hand-off tool SBAR on patient safety: a systematic review. *BMJ Open.* **8**,e022202.

Nursing and Midwifery Council (NMC) (2015). *The Code.* https://www.nmc.org.uk/globalassets/sitedocuments/nmc-publications/nmc-code.pdf (last accessed 16.1.2020).

Nursing and Midwifery Council (NMC) (2019). *Future nurse: Standards of proficiency of registered nurses.* https://www.nmc.org.uk/globalassets/sitedocuments/education-standards/future-nurse-proficiencies.pdf (last accessed 16.1.2020).

O'Daniel, M. & Rosenstein, A. (2008). 'Professional communication and team collaboration' in Hughes, R.G. (ed.) *Patient safety and quality: An evidence-based handbook for nurses.* Rockville, MD: Agency for Healthcare Research and Quality (US) https://www.ncbi.nlm.nih.gov/books/NBK2651/ (last accessed 16.1.2020).

Shannon, C.E. & Weaver, W. (1949). *A mathematical model of communication.* Urbana: University of Illinois Press.

Sheridan, D.J. & Julian, D.G. (2016). Achievements and limitations of evidence based medicine. *Journal of the American College of Cardiology.* **68**(2.),204–13.

Stickley, S. (2011). From SOLER to SURETY for effective non-verbal communication. *Nurse Education in Practice.* **11**(6) 395–98. https://doi.org/10.1016/j.nepr.2011.03.021 (last accessed 16.1.2020).

Watson, R. (2012). 'So you think you care?' in McSherry, W., McSherry, R. & Watson, R. (eds) *Care in nursing: Principles, values and skills.* pp. 3-14. Oxford: Oxford University Press.

5 Making a successful career of nursing

Introduction

As nursing is a profession that encompasses many areas of practice, potential nursing career pathways are many and various, depending on personal choice, the chosen area of practice and opportunities encountered. Although few people enter the profession with a predetermined career path, being a registered nurse can be a highly satisfying lifelong career, offering a great deal of variety, which enables the great nurse to fully utilise the skills of Hand, Heart and Head, as well as the underpinning, integral professional values that are transferable across the whole range of potential practice areas.

This chapter will explore some of these career opportunities, as well as identify some of the potential difficulties registered nurses may encounter along their career path, exploring how Hand, Heart and Head, counter-balanced by the self-care requirements of resilience and coping, can be combined to ensure the great nurse can have a successful lifelong career in nursing.

Initial career choices

In the nineteenth century and the first two-thirds of the twentieth century, an apprenticeship model of nurse training predominated in the UK. This began to change in the latter half of the twentieth century in response to the increased focus on nursing being recognised as a profession (Bradshaw 2001). An apprentice is usually someone who learns a trade from a skilled and experienced tradesperson (who is often their employer). The apprentice is paid a low wage for the contribution they make to the work they do. Until the 1970s, the model for nurse training often involved something similar – student nurses were recruited by specific employers, normally a hospital. As well as receiving some education from the employer's own school of nursing, they worked for a small wage, as part of the nursing team, and learnt mainly 'on the job' by working alongside others and, sometimes, unsupervised, with a very small number of nurses trained at graduate level by a few universities.

This model of nurse education has now been replaced in most countries by undergraduate nursing programmes, normally based at universities, where student nurses are full-time students rather than employees. This means one of the first choices an aspirant nurse has to make is which university to study at. It is important to note that, as a practice-based profession, modern nursing education still relies heavily on nursing students working alongside experienced qualified and educated practitioners. This means the student contribution to the workforce is carefully controlled and student nurses must always work under the supervision of a registered nurse or other qualified practitioner.

Once the future great nurse has chosen where to undertake their nursing education, they have to decide which type of nursing course they would like to undertake, and how best to achieve that choice. Internationally, there are many and varied routes to becoming a nurse and the specific choice of route may have a significant impact on future career opportunities. It is important to note that 'nurse' is not a protected professional title; anyone can call themselves a nurse, but not everyone who uses the title nurse will be on a professional register.

In most countries, there are many people called nurses who work at levels which normally require direct supervision by a registered nurse. In some countries, these nurses are likely to be regulated, which means they will have undertaken some form of structured education. In the UK, these are usually known as Nursing Associates, and they hold a form of registration with the Nursing and Midwifery Council (NMC). In the USA, they are known as Certified Nursing Assistants (CNAs) or Licenced Practical Nurses (LPNs), all of whom have lower levels of educational preparation for their role than a registered nurse. However, it is important to recognise that there is considerable international variation in the educational preparation of non-registered nurses.

Career opportunities for non-registered nurses are likely to be limited and the main option available is to undertake further education to gain registration. However, outside the UK possible routes to gaining registration are highly varied.

More commonly, people who want to undertake a career in nursing will enter an undergraduate degree programme which leads directly to registered nurse status upon successful completion. The opportunity to undertake a degree in nursing is available in many countries across the world and degree-level registered nurses are widely accepted as the standard for best practice. Some countries also offer opportunities for people who are already graduates in a range of subject areas to undertake postgraduate-level studies in nursing, also leading to professional registration.

Having decided to become a registered nurse, the next early career choice is deciding which type of nurse to become. In many countries there is little choice, as educational programmes all follow a similar training pathway, leading to a single type of general registration, with specialism only taking place after qualification. In the UK, there are four different routes to gaining registration and an early career choice is which of these to follow.

The four areas of nursing practice in the UK recognised by the NMC are:

- Adult nursing
- Children's nursing
- Learning disabilities nursing

● Mental health nursing.

These are known as fields of practice, and nurses who wish to gain registration in one of these fields will follow a specific educational programme focused on their chosen field. Opportunities to move between fields, either during a programme of study or following registration, can be limited so it is important that this early career choice is carefully thought through.

Learning activity 5.1 Your view of nursing

Nursing means many things to many people.

● Regardless of how long you have been a nurse, or how long you have wanted to be a nurse, what does nursing mean to you? What are the key elements of nursing that you are attracted to?

● Think about the ideas of Hand, Heart and Head. Are you more attracted to, or more comfortable with, different elements of these areas of nursing work? What personal qualities do you have that will make you a successful nurse?

● List: 1) Your top 5 ideas about what nursing means to you; 2) Your top 5 key reasons for being attracted to a career in nursing; 3) The top 5 qualities you have that will make you a successful nurse.

● Don't worry if there is some overlap. Instead, reflect on why nursing appeals to you. Is there a common thread and, if so, how can you use it to steer your career forward?

Early career choices

Although, at the pre-career stage, an aspirant registered nurse has already made several important decisions about their future career, a whole variety of further options become available once registration has been successfully gained. These may range from simply deciding where to take up a first post after qualification or focus on longer-term career ambitions.

Choice of first post following qualification is normally based on several factors, including personal preference for a particular clinical area, possibly based on previous experience, or a practice placement in that area. However, this may be constrained by the availability of jobs and the personal circumstances of the individual, which may necessitate taking some time out from work or study or relocating. Most newly qualified registered nurses seek to consolidate the skills learned in their nursing programme by spending a substantial period working in clinical practice. In most countries, including the UK, this consolidation of knowledge and skills is not mandatory and, although many employers offer preceptorship programmes, there is considerable variation in the support available. (For additional information on preceptorship, see Chapter 3.)

A newly qualified registered nurse may also start to think about their longer-term career ambitions, focusing on the different types of practice that might be available to, and appropriate, for them. The number of formal options varies widely internationally but, in the UK, there are a range of additional professional qualifications a registered nurse can gain following initial registration. Those that lead to additional registration are outlined in Table 5.1.

Table 5.1 Additional registerable professional qualifications

District nursing	District nurses commonly visit people in their own homes or run community-based clinics. They frequently work 1:1 with a range of people, generally focusing on physical care needs.
Health visiting	Health visitors normally work with families with children (from birth until around the age of 5). They are based in the community and may do a range of home visits or run clinics. They carry out a public health role and provide additional support for families with specific needs.
School nursing	School nurses are based within schools to support the health needs of school-age children, in collaboration with families and teachers. They can be involved in a mix of health screening, public health, disease management and child protection roles.
Occupational health nursing	Occupational health nurses are community based, normally with a specific employer, and offer a public health, disease management and work-based safety service for people in the workplace.

In the UK, there are a number of other options which lead to professionally recordable qualifications, including those listed in Table 5.2.

Box 5.1 Additional professional qualifications recordable with the NMC

- Community and independent prescriber
- Lecturer/Practice educator
- SPA: Specialist practitioner, Adult nursing
- SPMH: Specialist practitioner, Mental health
- SPC: Specialist practitioner, Children's nursing
- SPLD: Specialist practitioner, Learning disability nurse
- SPGP: Specialist practitioner, General practice nursing
- SCMH: Specialist practitioner, Community mental health nursing
- SCLD: Specialist practitioner, Community learning disabilities nursing
- SPCC: Specialist practitioner, Community children's nursing
- SPDN: Specialist practitioner, District nursing

For additional information, see: https://www.nmc.org.uk/registration/staying-on-the-register/your-statement-of-entry/registration-and-qualification-codes/

As well as qualifications which are professionally registrable or recordable, there is also a very wide range of additional qualifications a nurse can obtain which fall within the realm of Continuous Professional Development (CPD). CPD opportunities vary widely, from in-house training offered by specific employers, to more formal educational routes such as stand-alone modules, postgraduate certificates, diplomas and Masters' level programmes offered by higher-education providers. Choice of further CPD will be dependent on each nurse's chosen career path, the needs of their employer, and the opportunities and resources available to support their professional development. As discussed in Chapter 3, a successful nursing career involves continuous engagement with lifelong learning as a fundamental requirement of being a great nurse.

Learning activity 5.2 Your career goals

As a soon-to-be qualified or newly qualified nurse, it is not always easy to plan a career. In many ways, it's more useful to think about where you want to be at some point in the not-too-distant future, so think about a point five years from now.

- Where do you want to be in five years' time?
- Think about your personal and life goals as well as your career goals. Try writing a list of the things you would like to happen over that period of time.
- Once you have your list, try to prioritise the items. Not everyone is career orientated, and having a job which is personally satisfying can be as worthy a goal as scaling the career ladder, so this is a really good opportunity to think about what's important to you, and try to develop a sense of direction that will support you in moving towards that goal.

Later career choices

As great nurses progress across a working lifetime, their initial ideas and aspirations may change, either as a consequence of personal development or through changing workplace and patient needs. Many nurses therefore arrive at a stage in their careers when they feel the need to take stock, to think about what they have done already, the choices they have made and where they would like to go in the future.

Later career choices tend to focus on four key areas of nursing practice which bring the Hand, Heart and Head approach into clearer focus, with a different balance of these essential elements across the career pathway:

1. Advanced clinical practice
2. Leadership and management roles
3. Educational roles
4. Research roles.

Advanced clinical practice

Most people who decide to follow a career in nursing are drawn to it by a desire to work with people in some form of clinical practice. If working with patients and their families remains an important part of a nurse's role, developing a career in advanced clinical practice can be an excellent way of maintaining that contact, whilst working at a higher level than initial registration. Advanced clinical practice roles are available in many areas of nursing practice and across all specialist fields.

In the UK, the Royal College of Nursing (RCN 2018) defines advanced clinical practice in nursing as applying to those who are:

> 'educated at Master's Level in clinical practice and have been assessed as competent in practice using their expert clinical knowledge and skills. They have the freedom and authority to act, making autonomous decisions in the assessment, diagnosis and treatment of patients...'

It is important to note that, both in the UK and internationally, there is currently no clear or agreed definition of what an advanced clinical practitioner is, or what qualifications are needed to gain the title. The United States is one of the few countries where it is possible to register as an advanced registered nurse practitioner (ARNP) after undertaking additional specialised postgraduate education. However, the range of practitioners eligible for this level of registration is highly varied, including nurse midwives, clinical nurse specialists and nurse anaesthetists.

This lack of consensus has led to several divergent interpretations of the advanced clinical practice role, although there is a general consensus that it should contain the competency elements listed in Box 5.2 which are also known as 'pillars of practice' (RCN 2018).

Box 5.2 Pillars of practice for advanced clinical practice

1. Direct clinical practice
2. Leadership and collaborative practice
3. Education and learning
4. Research and evidence-based practice

When considering advanced clinical practice, key areas of competency may include those listed in Box 5.3.

Box 5.3 Advanced clinical practice competencies

1. Practise autonomously, using a person-centred approach, within the expanded scope of practice.

2. Demonstrate comprehensive skills for assessment, diagnosis, treatment, management and prescribing within the field of practice.

3. Use clinical judgement in managing complex and unpredictable care events, drawing upon an appropriate range of inter-agency and professional resources in their practice.

4. Demonstrate ability to manage and negotiate person-centred health-related/care needs for patients and their families.

5. Monitor and report quality issues affecting the provision of advanced nursing care delivery.

For leadership roles, the required competencies are listed in Box 5.4

Box 5.4 Leadership competencies

1. Develop and sustain partnerships and networks to influence and improve healthcare outcomes and healthcare delivery.
2. Engage stakeholders and use high-level negotiating and influencing skills to develop and improve practice, processes and systems.
3. Provide professional and clinical advice to colleagues regarding therapeutic interventions, practice and service improvement.
4. Demonstrate resilience as a clinical and professional leader.
5. Develop robust governance systems by interpreting and synthesising information from a variety of sources, in order to contribute to the development and implementation of evidence-based protocols, documentation processes, standards, policies and clinical guidelines, and promote their use in practice.

Competencies for lifelong learning and educational needs include those listed in Box 5.5.

Box 5.5 Lifelong learning competencies

1. Continue to keep knowledge and skills up to date by engaging in a range of relevant learning and development activities.
2. Educate, supervise or mentor nursing colleagues and others in the healthcare team.
3. Advocate and contribute to the development of an organisational culture that supports continuous learning and development, evidence-based practice and succession planning.
4. Lead person-centred care using a practice development approach.
5. Lead and contribute to a range of audit and evaluation strategies which inform education and learning.

Finally, the competencies required for evidence-based practice are listed in Box 5.6.

Box 5.6 Evidence-based practice competencies

1. Contribute to and undertake activities, including research, that monitor and improve the quality of healthcare and the effectiveness of practice.
2. Critically appraise the outcomes of relevant research and evaluations and apply the information to improve practice.
3. Advocate and contribute to the development of a research culture that supports evidence-based practice.
4. Lead and contribute to publications and dissemination of work.
5. Demonstrate understanding and application of a range of research methodologies.

Boxes 5.2 to 5.6 are all taken from: Department of Health, Social Services and Public Safety 2016.

Although these competencies seem comprehensive, several variations exist and not all of them are applicable to every situation or role. The lack of agreed definition for advanced clinical practice also means that there is an abundance of role titles and different routes for practitioners to follow. Common role titles include: nurse consultant, clinical nurse specialist, advanced nurse practitioner and specialist nurse practitioner.

When considering developing a career path towards advanced clinical practice, it is important for the nurse to plan this carefully. Many of the roles are specific to an employing organisation and decisions about role opportunities and the required education/training for them may need to be taken in consultation with that role provider. Some roles include the need for carefully planned clinical supervision or mentorship and there may be limited availability of suitable supervisors and mentors. Several higher-education providers offer a wide range of advanced clinical practice programmes, and successful completion of one of these programmes may also offer a route into advanced clinical practice. Again, the nurse needs to make a careful choice about which programme is most suitable for their chosen career.

Leadership and management roles

Although leadership/management is included as one of the four competency elements or pillars of advanced practice, it is also possible to follow a career in leadership and management without following an advanced clinical practice route. If you would like to know more about the different types of leaders, as well as the different theories of management and leadership, there is a fuller discussion of those in Chapter 6. In this section, the key focus is on leadership and management as a possible later career choice.

Leadership within healthcare is commonly regarded as one of the most important elements in ensuring the delivery of high-quality healthcare services (King's Fund 2015) through its fundamental role in shaping healthcare culture and the behaviours of those in leadership roles. Jane Cummings (2014), the Chief Nurse for England, highlighted the almost natural ability of great nurses to assume leadership roles from the earliest stages in their careers, making decisions about patient care, and supervising those working under them, in specific leadership roles such as staff nurses and ward managers.

The importance of excellent leadership within healthcare is reflected by the prioritisation of leadership skills and training within healthcare services, including (in the UK) the development of the NHS Leadership training academy (for further information see: https://www.leadershipacademy. nhs.uk/programmes/) which offers a broad range of leadership programmes, from ward manager level to aspiring chief executives.

The priorities for leadership within nursing and healthcare are numerous and highly varied, resulting in a wide choice of possible career routes. However, there are some clear commonalities between leadership roles, regardless of their specific healthcare context.

Storey and Holti (2013) suggest leadership should focus on three key elements:

1. Provide and justify a clear sense of purpose and contribution for staff

2. Motivate teams and individuals to work effectively

3. Focus on improving system performance.

Meanwhile, the NHS Leadership Academy (2014) works within a bespoke leadership framework comprising nine different elements:

1. Inspiring shared purpose

2. Leading with care

3. Evaluating information

4. Connecting our service

5. Sharing the vision

6. Engaging the team

7. Holding to account

8. Developing capability

9. Influencing for results.

Within this NHS leadership model, each of the nine elements can be individually assessed as: essential, proficient, strong and exemplary. To take the first element as an example, when seeking to 'inspire shared purpose', it would be:

● Essential – to demonstrate an ability to stay true to NHS values

● Proficient – to hold on to those principles under pressure

● Strong – to take a personal risk to stand up for a shared purpose

● Exemplary – to focus on the individual leader making courageous challenges for the benefit of the service.

This type of leadership framework approach is adaptable to many leadership situations, and is also designed to provide flexibility in the ever-changing world of healthcare provision, as well as supporting nurse leaders in the essential requirement of working collaboratively within their own profession and with other healthcare professionals, as well as with their patients and service users.

In common with advanced clinical practice roles, there is no clear definition of what makes a nurse leader. Nurse leadership may take the form of someone with a designated leadership title, such as chief nurse, matron, ward manager, or – more simply – it may be someone others turn towards to lead the way in times of crisis or indecision. Career planning for management roles can be difficult, as there is no one route forward. It therefore needs to be done in collaboration with an employer and may be dependent on the particular job and educational opportunities that are available. Education opportunities in leadership are also provided by a range of higher-education institutions (HEIs) but, again, careful choice is essential to find the one which is best suited to the individual's career aspirations and circumstances.

Educational roles

As well as being naturally positioned to take up leadership roles, many great nurses are equally well placed to move into roles with a more educational focus, either within the healthcare environment or by moving into the educational sector. Nurses naturally have the skills needed to work as role models for others. Their roles as mentors and preceptors (see Chapters 3 and 6) also place them in an excellent position to make later career choices taking them into a more defined educational role that involves facilitating the learning of others and inspiring them to be great nurses too. From their experience in health education and health promotion activities, nurses have many directly transferable communication skills designed to facilitate the transfer of knowledge and acquisition of learning as well as consequent behaviour change, all of which are directly applicable to an educational career.

Career frameworks for following an educational route are less well developed than those of advanced clinical practice or leadership. Although there is no specific framework available at present, educational roles normally follow one of two routes in the UK: those who work in educational roles with a clinical healthcare provider and have a specific remit focused on the individual employer's requirements; and those who leave clinical practice to undertake an educational career normally within the higher-education sector.

For those nurses interested in working in an educational role, moving into a post with either an element of educational input or a sole focus on education for staff within clinical practice can be their first move towards an education career path. Types of roles which are currently available in the UK may include: practice education facilitators, practice educators and clinical educators. However, in common with other career options, actual titles and role descriptions can vary from one employing organisation to another.

Nurses wishing to follow a career in the educational sector (away from direct clinical practice) will commonly find that their career choices involve moving to a role with a higher-education institution (HEI) such as a university or a further-education institution (FEI) such as a college. The requirements for clinical staff seeking a change of career, and wanting to move into education, again vary between employing organisations but would normally require a nurse to have undertaken a substantial period of clinical practice, and to have achieved a high level of experience and seniority in their clinical role. They may also have a range of directly transferable educational experiences, either in an advanced clinical practice role, or a combined educational and practice role, and normally they should also have achieved a higher level of specialist clinical/academic qualification such as a postgraduate award at Master's level.

Internationally, pre-registration nurse education mainly takes place in the higher-education sector with registration only attainable at degree level, meaning that nurse educators must have the necessary academic and learning facilitation skills and advanced knowledge base to support the development of future generations of registered nurses. Aside from professional knowledge and expertise, nurses working in roles which are educationally focused will also need to demonstrate an ability to 'teach'. Most nurses working in this area will therefore need to undertake a specific educational qualification at the level of postgraduate certificate or postgraduate diploma. In the UK, they will also be expected to obtain a qualification that enables them to register an additional professionally recordable qualification in education with the NMC.

Once they have successfully obtained an educational post, most nurse educators will follow the same career trajectory as other academics in higher education; regardless of their area of expertise, this normally means following a path from lecturer to senior lecturer/principal lecturer, then reader and professor. Progression on this pathway is not automatic and, as with all other areas of nursing practice, requires a nurse educator to continue their ongoing lifelong educational pathway, undertaking more formal education which may include postgraduate studies at doctoral level and direct involvement in research. They will also need to undertake scholarly activities such as publication, conference presentation and project work, which generate more knowledge about their subject areas, as well as educational developments to support and improve students' experiences and learning.

Research roles

As with all later career roles, progression into a research-focused career pathway has no direct route, and no clearly outlined professional definition or level of registration. Many nurses who find themselves working directly in a research role may therefore have had a varied and circuitous route towards this position. However, many nurses working in research roles share a desire to change and improve nursing care, to find out more about their areas of knowledge and, ultimately, to develop knowledge that improves patient care and long-term patient outcomes.

Registered nurses already hold a range of transferable skills which are directly applicable to working in research roles: the ability to communicate clearly both verbally and in writing, good organisational skills, team working and, in some instances, the ability to work with data and technology. Traditionally, the global approach to formal research training consists of further academic study at postgraduate level, undertaking a Master's level qualification or doctoral-level study, either as a taught doctorate or a research doctorate. However, depending on the actual research role a nurse is undertaking, academic requirements can vary.

Within clinical practice, a nurse can undertake research roles in a variety of settings, working as a research nurse as part of a team involved in a larger-scale research project or trial. This may involve taking responsibility for elements of the research project, such as recruiting participants, checking eligibility, gaining consent, collecting data by performing specific tests such as taking blood samples or other observations, and obtaining information through interviews and questionnaires, as well as entering and analysing data. The research nurse's actual involvement is likely to vary, depending on each project and its specific requirements. The role may also be time-limited, according to the timespan allowed for each project.

Nurses who work in the field of clinical research, supporting individual projects and trials, will need many skills; and job security, isolation from clinical colleagues and career development can all be issues.

In the UK, the National Institute for Health Research (NIHR) not only provides support for nurses to undertake such roles and develop careers within clinical research, but has also developed its own strategy which stresses the importance and real impact on clinical practice improvements that can be provided by nurses working in clinical research areas (NIHR 2017). This strategy aims to:

1. Improve awareness and understanding of the specialty of clinical research nursing and its contribution and impact
2. Develop leaders to share best clinical research nursing practice locally, nationally and internationally
3. Promote innovation in research delivery practice to include the use of digital technologies to improve data quality and enable novel ways of using resources
4. Create a clinical research culture that is patient and public focused.

Awareness of the importance of clinical research has also led to the development of what are now known in the UK as Clinical Academic Career Pathways (CACPs). These have expanded from previously medically orientated roles to cover a whole range of nursing and allied healthcare professionals (Health Education England (HEE) 2018). As a joint initiative between the NIHR and HEE, this career framework offers support and funding for the following five steps into a future clinical academic career:

1. Internships
2. Pre-doctoral clinical academic fellowships
3. Clinical doctoral research fellowships
4. Clinical lectureships
5. Senior clinical lectureships.

It is anticipated that this approach will lead to improvements in research and innovation which will directly benefit patients as well as improving cost-effectiveness. Importantly, it will also develop nurses at a level of educational excellence to facilitate their development as future leaders across a range of clinical specialisms and healthcare research fields.

Research roles for nurses also exist in the educational sector and many nurses who move into a later career in education may also find themselves engaged in research activities, through undertaking their own doctoral studies, or by supporting other doctoral students to achieve their own research goals, or through collaboration in and leadership of research proposals and grant bids, resulting in extensive research projects. Much research activity in the educational sector is carried out in collaboration with national and international clinical colleagues, which can lead to considerable overlap between nurses working in research roles in the clinical and educational sectors as well as blurring of boundaries and responsibilities in large clinical trials between educational and clinical collaborators.

This collaborative approach can have many benefits for nurses who seek roles in research, providing change and flexibility, and the ability to work across a variety of teams and sectors. It may ultimately lead to senior research leadership roles that support real developments in nursing knowledge and practice with profound impacts on patient care and outcomes.

Learning activity 5.3 Your career route

- What is the right career route for you?
- Write a list of the 10 things you enjoy most about your nursing role, then the 10 things you find the least satisfying.
- What do your lists say about you?
- Do you enjoy hands-on patient care, or do you get more satisfaction from other aspects of your role?
- Do you have advanced organisational skills? Do you have a thirst for knowledge and a desire to create more knowledge? Or are you most satisfied by supporting learning in others?

Think about your lists. From these, it may become clear that your later career choices are focused in one area. If that is the case, now might be the time to start planning a career move.

This is also a good time to think about what you need to know about your chosen career path:

- What experience and qualifications are you likely to need?
- Where can you find the information you need?
- Who can you speak to?
- What sort of timeframe are you looking at?

This is a great opportunity to ask some of these questions and find the answers.

For some nurses, some or all of these elements are important. If that's the case for you, don't worry. Career choices can't be forced and one of the great joys of a successful career in nursing, and lifelong learning, is that movement in one career direction doesn't preclude future change.

Developing resilience and coping mechanisms

A significant aspect of having a long and successful career in nursing, in any of the roles discussed above, is the ability of each nurse to sustain their career and avoid being burnt out before they can reach their career goals. This is also an important issue in ensuring that the great nurse is able to maintain their 'head, heart and hand' approach as their career progresses and stay sufficiently motivated to make a difference to the lives of others.

It is obvious from the discussion so far in this book that nursing is a rewarding profession, but it is also clear that nurses face challenges every day as they witness human suffering and experience the 'emotional labour' of their role (see Chapter 2). For this reason, the concept of 'resilience' has become a cornerstone of nurses' career development.

Without the skills, resources and support to manage emotionally and physically demanding situations, nurses' health and well-being is likely to be threatened. Resilience is the inherent personal capacity that helps individual nurses deal with the adversities and demands they experience (Hart, Brannan & De Chesnay 2014). It includes the ability to successfully adapt to adversity (Delgado *et al.* 2017), along with the ability to recover and rebound from challenging situations that are often described as 'having a bad day'. It is also important for nurses to be able to learn from and grow stronger through difficult experiences (Thomas & Asselin 2018). Because of the pressured nature of much nursing practice, resilience is needed in everyday practice situations as well as when more unusual events occur. This is equally true for the novice nurse, the experienced or advanced practitioner, the leader, the educator and the researcher.

Some nurses are naturally more resilient than others. Having the type of character that is naturally better able to cope with adversity is thought to help – although resilience may also cause the individual to mask their distress and deal with it ineffectively, leading to problems later. Helping nurses to develop their resilience and coping skills, especially early in their careers, can make a difference to their experiences during their career and help them maintain the values of great nurses throughout.

The literature to date has mainly considered building resilience in student nurses, although it remains an important skill which can be developed throughout a nurse's career. Resilience training focuses on improving the self-care, self-efficacy, and work/life balance of individual nurses, with a view to reducing burnout. It tends to focus on adaptive skills and reflection on positive influences. One of the recognised barriers to building resilience is a culture that encourages nurses to be 'selfless'. This often means that nurses focus on taking care of others rather than themselves (Taylor 2019), leading to a lack of self-care that is incompatible with resilience.

Various methods to help build resilience are discussed in the literature. For example:

- **Increasing self-efficacy** – believing in oneself and taking control, rather than passively allowing things to happen
- **Developing coping skills** – learning about useful thoughts and actions in stressful situations
- **Seeking support** – working in teams in which members actively support one another and, additionally, seeking support outside a team through coaching, clinical supervision or mentorship (see Chapter 6)
- **Reflecting** – using the reflective process (see Chapter 3) to gain greater understanding of situations
- **Improving life/work balance and self-care** – recognising the need to have time to relax and take care of one's own physical and emotional needs and putting this into action.

Learning activity 5.4 Building resilience throughout your career

The Royal College of Nursing (RCN) in the UK has provided free access to a series of articles and other resources designed to help you to manage stress and build resilience. You don't have to be a member of the RCN to read the articles.

You can access the articles at the following link:

https://rcni.com/features/resources-managing-stress-and-building-resilience-79261

- Read two or three that catch your interest
- Identify some options in the articles that you can use to build on your own resilience and make a plan to put them into action.

Conclusion

Nursing is an amazing profession full of wonderful people with fulfilling and successful careers. A career in nursing offers numerous, constantly evolving opportunities, and great nurses are in a prime position to undertake a highly successful lifelong career journey. This flexibility and range of choice makes it likely that every great nurse's career will be different; and the opportunity to use the skills of 'hand, heart and head' is present in all aspects of nursing practice. Nursing is not an easy occupation to choose. Working with people in a range of difficult and potentially disturbing and stressful situations is far from straightforward and nurses do need to remember that self-care is an essential component of their career progression. Being resilient, and developing the skills needed to cope with the wide range of circumstances and people nurses encounter on a daily basis, are as vital to a successful career as any amount of forward planning. Ultimately, this combination enables nurses to demonstrate the great range of skills they possess and to successfully use them as they move forward to fulfil their own career aspirations.

The key points in this chapter can best be summarised in five steps that are essential to make a successful career of nursing – see Box 5.7.

Box 5.7 Steps to making a successful career of nursing

1. Think seriously about what initial career route is best for you.
2. Think about your personal preferences regarding your long-term career direction, and how they match your circumstances, skills and attributes.
3. Ensure you make informed decisions about what choices are available to you.
4. Take deliberate steps to protect yourself from burnout by taking care of your own needs and developing resilience.
5. Remember to enjoy your career – personal satisfaction is an essential element of a successful career as great nurse.

References

Bradshaw, A. (2001). *The nurse apprentice*. 1860–1977. London: Routledge.

Cummings, J. (2014). Blog. https://www.england.nhs.uk/blog/leadership-jane-cummings/ (last accessed 20.1.2020).

Delgado, C., Upton, D., Ranse, K., Furness T. & Foster, K. (2017). Nurses' resilience and the emotional labour of nursing work: An integrative review of empirical literature. *International Journal of Nursing Studies*. **70**, 71–88.

Department of Health and Social Care (2016). *Nursing Degree Apprenticeships Factsheet*. https://www.gov.uk/government/publications/nursing-degree-apprenticeships-factsheet/nursing-degree-apprenticeship-factsheet (last accessed 20.1.2020).

Department of Health, Social Services and Public Safety (2016). *Advanced Nursing Practice Framework*. https://www.health-ni.gov.uk/sites/default/files/publications/health/advanced-nursing-practice-framework.pdf (last accessed 20.1.2020).

Hart, P., Brannan, J. & De Chesnay, M. (2014). Resilience in nurses: an integrative review. *Journal of Nursing Management*. **22**(6), 720–734.

Health Education England (HEE) (2018). *Clinical Academic Career Framework*. https://www.hee.nhs.uk/sites/default/files/documents/2018-02%20CAC%20Framework.pdf (last accessed 20.1.2020).

The King's Fund (2015). *Leadership and Leadership Development in Healthcare*. https://www.kingsfund.org.uk/sites/default/files/field/field_publication_file/leadership-leadership-development-health-care-feb-2015.pdf (last accessed 20.1.2020).

National Institute for Health Research (NIHR) (2017). *Clinical Research Strategy*. https://www.nihr.ac.uk/documents/nihr-clinical-research-nurse-strategy-2017-2020/11501

NHS (2019). *Health Careers*. https://www.healthcareers.nhs.uk/explore-roles/nursing-careers (last accessed 20.1.2020).

NHS Leadership Academy (2014). *Healthcare leadership model*. https://www.leadershipacademy.nhs.uk/resources/healthcare-leadership-model/ (last accessed 20.1.2020).

Nursing and Midwifery Council (NMC) (2019a). *Becoming a nurse, midwife or nursing associate*. https://www.nmc.org.uk/education/becoming-a-nurse-midwife-nursing-associate/ (last accessed 20.1.2020).

Nursing and Midwifery Council (NMC) (2019b). *Registration*. https://www.nmc.org.uk/registration/staying-on-the-register/your-statement-of-entry/registration-and-qualification-codes/ (last accessed 20.1.2020).

Royal College of Nursing (RCN) (2018). *Advanced Practice Standards*. https://www.rcn.org.uk/professional-development/advanced-practice-standards (last accessed 20.1.2020).

Royal College of Nursing (RCN) (2019). *Career Ideas and Inspiration*. https://www.rcn.org.uk/professional-development/your-career/nurse/career-crossroads/career-ideas-and-inspiration (last accessed 20.1.2020).

Storey, J. & Holti, R. (2013). *Towards a new model of leadership for the NHS*. https://www.leadershipacademy.nhs.uk/wp-content/uploads/2013/05/Towards-a-New-Model-of-Leadership-2013.pdf (last accessed 20.1.2020).

Taylor, R. (2019). Contemporary issues: Resilience training alone is an incomplete intervention. *Nurse Education Today*. **78**, 10–13.

Thomas, L. & Asselin, M. (2018). Promoting resilience among nursing students in clinical education. *Nurse Education in Practice*. **28**, 231–34.

Chapter 6

Supporting and influencing others to be great nurses

Introduction

Nursing skill and practice are not static, and great nurses continue to learn and develop throughout their careers so that they are always able to provide the best care, based on up-to-date knowledge and evidence. As discussed in Chapters 3 and 4, learning is not only for those aspiring to be registered nurses, but for registered nurses themselves – as their careers progress and their skills, competence and expertise develop. Nurses almost always work in teams and, importantly, each team member has collective responsibility for the education and development both of themselves and of other nurses in the team, before and after registration. Hence, every great nurse needs the knowledge, skills and attitudes needed to ensure that those around them are educated and supported in their practice in a way that enables them to give the best care. By the same token, an essential part of every great nurse's role is to support the learning and development of those with whom they work, in a spirit of mutual respect and collaboration. This is evident from the 'Sharing skills and knowledge and supporting the learning of others' section of *The Code* (NMC 2015), as shown in Box 6.1.

This chapter aims to explore the ways in which nurses can support others in their team and wider work community to develop and improve their practice so that they can meet their own aspirations and strive to be great nurses with the job satisfaction that comes from that. Continuous education and professional development in nursing can be facilitated by nurses themselves so this chapter will consider the best approaches to profession-led education and development of all nurses. Throughout the chapter the term 'learner' will be used to refer to any nurse who is engaged in learning.

Box 6.1 Sharing skills and knowledge and supporting the learning of others

The Code (NMC 2015) often refers to the need to learn and support the learning of others. Specifically, it states (on p.10) that nurses should:

9.1 Provide honest, accurate and constructive feedback to colleagues

9.2 Gather and reflect on feedback from a variety of sources, using it to improve your practice and performance

9.3 Deal with differences of professional opinion with colleagues by discussion and informed debate, respecting their views and opinions and behaving in a professional way at all times

9.4 Support students' and colleagues' learning to help them develop their professional competence and confidence.

Learning activity 6.1 Supporting the learning and development of others

Consider the section of *The Code* concerning 'Sharing skills and knowledge and supporting the learning of others' outlined in Box 6.1 above.

Identify two events from your recent practice:

1. Where someone else shared their knowledge and/or skills with you

2. Where you shared your knowledge and/or skills with someone else.

Think about your experiences of both these events.

In what ways did they emulate the NMC *Code* (above), in relation to your learning and supporting the learning of others?

What made these experiences more positive and what made them less positive?

How do these experiences illustrate how great nursing can develop?

How can the head, heart and hand principles be applied to sharing knowledge and skills?

Continuing professional development

As discussed briefly in Chapter 3, continuing professional development (CPD) is central to being a great nurse. It is the means by which nurses ensure that their knowledge and skills are up to date and that they are competent/proficient in providing nursing care. CPD is linked with lifelong learning, recognising that learning must continue to take place throughout a nurse's career so that care can be safe and effective. CPD is also instrumental in career progression for nurses, as well as job satisfaction, and in the retention of nurses in the profession or with an employer (Drey *et al.* 2009). In the UK, the need for continuing learning is enshrined in the NMC's revalidation process which expects nurses to undertake a minimum of 35 hours' CPD over three years and to provide evidence of learning (see http://revalidation.nmc.org.uk/) with the aim of ensuring that they continue to grow and develop as great nurses using the head, heart and hand.

Working in a culture where CPD is part of everyone's working life is essential in order to develop great nursing teams. The range of learning opportunities for CPD can vary, from planned educational provision (such as formal courses) to less formal approaches (such as individual study through reading and reflective and experiential learning). Some areas of practice are recognised as being so fundamental to patient safety and effective care that attendance at CPD activities is mandatory. This typically includes topics such as infection prevention, health and safety, vulnerable child and adult protection and emergency procedures. Failure to attend such training activities can lead to disciplinary action, but even this may not mean that attendance at mandatory CPD sessions has a positive impact on practice, or even that much is learned. Learners must actively apply what they have learned to their practice. Attending conferences and study days and engaging in practice networks and communities of practice are other ways to further professional knowledge and skills.

The impact of CPD activity on professional practice and positive change is often uncertain, as it is difficult to evaluate its impact on care delivery. The characteristics of the individual practitioner, including their motivation and readiness to learn, and to influence practice, probably play a significant part in the practical impact of their CPD (Lee 2011). An approach is needed which ensures that practice benefit is achieved at an individual, team and organisational level across all elements of 'hand, heart and head' (Manley *et al.* 2018).

The clinical settings where patient care takes place are also important learning environments for everyone involved in providing and supporting great care. The culture and environment of learning in any given clinical setting can significantly influence the climate of continuing learning and development for nurses and other health professionals who work there. A culture in which skills and knowledge are passed on to others as a natural part of clinical practice is a feature of settings where great nurses work. Supporting others in gaining expertise, experience and knowledge is central to ensuring consistently excellent care.

A management and leadership culture that supports continuous learning and development for all members of staff also supports great healthcare practice. Organisations that support staff in attending learning events, and provide opportunities for learning in the workplace, as well as supporting the development of practice based on learning (even when staff resources are under pressure) are the organisations most likely to deliver the best care.

Approaches to supporting clinical learning for others

Clinical supervision, mentoring and coaching are terms that are commonly applied to supporting the learning of others in the nursing profession; and these terms are broadly defined in Box 6.2. In all these approaches, the focus tends to be on helping others to learn, rather than simply 'teaching' them; most people learn more from being actively engaged in learning, rather than being told what is right by a 'teacher'. Great mentors, clinical supervisors and coaches are widely considered to have a positive impact on the learning, skills, behaviours and attitudes of others.

Box 6.2 Definitions of mentoring, clinical supervision and coaching

Mentoring

In the nursing profession, mentoring has traditionally been applied to the relationship between nursing students and their practice supervisors. Definitions tend to include: giving support; providing assistance and guidance in learning; helping to develop skills, behaviours and attitudes; stimulating reflection; promoting learning; reducing stress in clinical practice; bridging the theory-practice gap and acting as a role model (Huybrecht *et al.* 2011). Often, a mentor is also the person who undertakes practice assessment of students' performance. Recently, the term 'practice supervisor' has become more popular when discussing this relationship. Mentorship is a term commonly used in other workplaces outside healthcare. It has a broader definition that focuses on learning support for someone as part of their everyday work.

Clinical supervision

Clinical supervision tends to be more focused on the development of clinical practice in qualified nurses. It is a process that is broadly linked to creating a relationship between a clinical supervisor and supervisee that aims to create a supportive, collaborative environment in which participants have an opportunity to discuss and reflect on their practice and develop their own great clinical practice through mutual support and peer learning (Cummins 2009). Clinical supervision has traditionally been focused on the new graduate nurse and has now been largely superseded by the term 'coaching' applied to clinical practice.

Coaching

Coaching is still a relatively new term applied to nursing education. It tends to involve a partnership between a coach and coachee that involves creative discussion to enable development of the individual. Mutually understood goals and objectives, focused on personal and professional development needs, are identified and these motivate the coachee toward higher-level practice (Tee, Jowett & Bechelet-Carter 2009). Coaching is considered in more detail in the following section.

Coaching

As discussed in Chapters 3 and 4, nurses learn most of their craft from other nurses and health practitioners in the real world of everyday practice so that they can develop competence/proficiency in the range of diverse clinical skills. This continues once the nurse is a registered practitioner and also applies to those in caring roles other than registered nurses, such as nursing assistants and associate nurses.

Learning through real-life experiences that reflect the nurse's present and future practice is often referred to as 'situated learning' (Stalmeijer *et al.* 2009); and the 'cognitive apprenticeship model' (Collins, Brown & Newman 1989) is often applied to clinical education in nursing. This suggests that the best clinical learning takes place when the thinking processes used in the practice of complex skills are part of the learning experience. Working with proficient and expert practitioners (themselves great nurses) can help less experienced nurses to learn by observing expert practice and then undertaking clinical interventions with support and supervision as well as developing insight into the cognitive processes needed to practise effectively at a more advanced level. Collins, Brown & Newman (1989) proposed six approaches to facilitating the learning of others in clinical situations:

- **Coaching** – observing learners and providing feedback on their performance
- **Scaffolding** – providing support tailored to learners' individual knowledge levels (this support is gradually reduced and eventually withdrawn)
- **Articulation** – questioning learners and stimulating the learners' own questions
- **Reflection** – stimulating learners to look back on and evaluate their performance
- **Exploration** – encouraging learners to devise and work towards their own personal learning goals.

Recently, coaching has become an increasingly popular method for helping others to learn and develop. It is associated with facilitation – a process of helping others to achieve but without getting directly involved. Whitmore (2017) defines coaching as: '…helping someone to unlock their potential to maximize their own performance'. In nursing, coaching is increasingly identified as an effective approach to promoting learning and developing self-awareness in others (Kelton 2014). It is also suggested as a way to promote patient safety and develop resilience in nurses by helping them develop capability and competence (Duff 2013).

Great coaches have the qualities, skills and values discussed in Chapters 2 and 4. They often act as role models for other practitioners: embodying great nursing to set an example to others and enabling others to learn from them. Whitmore (2017) suggests that good coaches are emotionally intelligent and can bring out emotional intelligence in others. Elements of coaching include: an interactive and interpersonal process, supporting others to develop professional practice, career development and acquisition of skills, improving competence and confidence in others and improving work satisfaction. The best coaches tend to be those with extensive experience of practice. They are advanced or expert practitioners who can support others in developing their skills and applying theoretical knowledge to develop great nursing practice (Kowalski & Casper 2007). Many great nurses are often naturally good coaches and coach others without necessarily realising that they are coaching. Coaching is also an integral part of patient education, support and health improvement so these skills are also used in a clinical context.

Learning to coach effectively is increasingly seen as a way to develop your skills in supporting the learning of others. Learning some of the principles and methods of coaching can be a useful way to develop coaching skills. Coaching is an approach commonly used in business and sport, where its principles have developed. The guiding principles of coaching include:

- Showing respect to the coachee (or learner)
- Seeking to develop their potential
- Communicating effectively
- Providing specific feedback
- Using goal setting to motivate and provide appropriate challenges.

(Taken from: Kelton 2014)

These coaching principles can be used in many situations. This might include informal coaching where the coach and coachee are working together clinically and coaching takes place as a natural part of the clinical event. Coaching sessions can also be formalised, and specific time set aside to work on a specific goal. A commonly used coaching model is the GROW model devised by Whitmore (2017) that can be used to structure both informal and informal coaching (see Figure 6.1). The model offers four steps to help the coach to structure the coaching relationship, event or session. These stages can help the coach to support the coachee in understanding their own aspirations, articulating their current situation and beliefs, identifying what resources and possibilities are available to them and what actions they might need to take to achieve their goals.

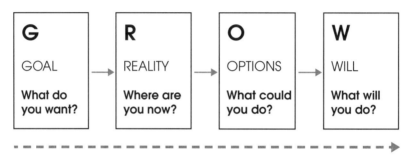

Figure 6.1 The GROW model of coaching (Whitmore 2017)

Leadership

Leadership is another important aspect of supporting others in striving to be great nurses, to create a culture that supports continuous professional development and enhanced patient care. The importance of leadership in nursing practice and its impact on the quality of patient care was identified in Chapter 5 – leadership is one of the many attributes that enables great nurses to deliver the best nursing care and support others to do the same. However, although the importance of good leadership is easy to recognise, it is more difficult to determine what constitutes good leadership, with different needs for different situations, as well as a diverse range of leadership approaches and models. This section will identify some of the different approaches to leadership and briefly consider which may be the most useful to support great nursing practice.

According to the King's Fund (2015), the three key tasks of a leader are to provide:

1. **Direction** – ensuring agreement
2. **Alignment** – ensuring effective coordination and integration
3. **Commitment** – taking personal responsibility to ensure organisational success.

Within healthcare, these tasks are focused on providing safe, high-quality compassionate care, using 'hand, head and heart'. In order to demonstrate excellence in these leadership tasks, the nurse leader must also be supportive, empathetic and use a leadership style which supports learning and seeks the active collaboration of other staff, and those patients receiving care. Clear lines of communication are essential, allowing both positive and negative feedback and a transparent process for dealing with any issues (such as poor performance) as soon as they arise.

There is some debate in the multi-professional leadership literature on whether leadership skills can be taught, or whether they simply occur naturally within some individuals (Echevarria, Patterson & Krouse 2017). It is clear that some personality traits make people more effective leaders than others. The eight key personality characteristics can be summarised as:

1. High energy levels and stress tolerance – stamina
2. Self-confidence
3. An internal locus of control – they believe they can exert control over external events
4. Emotional maturity
5. Personal integrity
6. Socialised power motivation – seeking power to improve
7. Achievement orientation
8. Low need for affiliation – not needing to be liked.

(Taken from: Yukl 2013)

Learning activity 6.2 Your leadership skills and qualities

It is highly unlikely one individual will possess all eight of the personality characteristics Yukl (2013) has suggested (see above) which contribute to making a good leader.

- Which of those characteristics do you think you possess?
- Which of those characteristics do you think you need help with?
- If you are not sure, why not ask a friend or colleague?

Having some insight into your own abilities can be really helpful. For instance, if you have high energy levels but lower self-confidence, you could start to look at how you could improve your self-confidence and develop your own leadership skills. Think about identifying a leadership coach to help you do this.

Several theories of leadership have been proposed that aim to identify the most effective leadership approaches, as well as offering models that can be used to encourage effective leadership development. Within healthcare, the two most commonly identified approaches to leadership are known as the 'transactional approach' and the 'transformational approach' (King's Fund 2015).

The transactional approach to leadership, first suggested by Bass (1998), encapsulates what may be considered the more traditional approach to management rather than leadership. Transactional leaders work at the level of transactions; they identify issues or tasks which need to be dealt with, they allot work, control resources, information and data and monitor performance of those tasks. Although this approach may be useful in dealing with the day-to-day issues that arise in many areas of nurses' work, it clearly has some disadvantages as a leadership style. These disadvantages include an ongoing focus on task monitoring, which can be perceived negatively; and a failure to work collaboratively and transparently with other members of the team, which can lead to a lack of team empowerment and engagement.

Transformational leadership, in contrast, has a wider scope. Transformational leaders are focused on bigger issues and may have a vision for the future that includes the proactive pursuit of change both for individuals and the organisations in which they work. Transformational leaders may have a more complex relationship with their staff, but this can be an advantage in terms of helping to build effective long-term relationships between team members united in a common purpose, as well as improving individual levels of work satisfaction amongst those team members. (To find out more about leadership styles, you could look at: Frankel 2011, Spence Laschinger *et al.* 2011, Mossiani, Bagnasco & Sasso 2017.) Ultimately, the aim of the transformational leader is to motivate those who work for them to accomplish more than they might otherwise have done.

One of the key attributes of great nurses, as discussed in Chapter 2, is that they embrace the values required to have compassion for others, linked to an understanding of what comprises emotionally intelligent behaviour and decision-making (the use of the heart). Transformational leadership aligns positively with these key nursing skills through the use of the heart, by adopting an emotionally intelligent approach to leadership and, ultimately, staff motivation and development. It also uses the hand and head, to demonstrate skills of organisation, delegation and feedback.

Recognition of the importance of the transformational leadership approach (with its inherent rejection of the much narrower managerial transactional approach) has led directly to recognition of the inherent value of a related leadership model known as 'servant leadership' where the primary focus is on the essential element of relationship building within a leadership context (Fahlberg & Toomey 2016). Leaders who adopt the servant leader approach follow five key practices. They:

1. Develop a vision

2. Listen and learn before acting

3. Invest in others

4. Give away power – allow others a voice

5. Work to build a collaborative community.

When seeking to improve nursing care, aiming towards excellence at both the individual and collective level, servant leadership encapsulates many of the nursing values which lead to great practice and support the learning and development of others. As well as offering nurse leaders a tool to challenge and manage poor practice in a responsible and positive manner, servant leadership also ensures that great nurse leaders can use emotional intelligence to provide the support needed to encourage and empower all nurses to deliver the best possible nursing care.

Managing performance and challenging poor practice

It is essential to recognise that nurses have a significant influence on patient experiences and outcomes. The goal of great nursing is to provide excellent care 100% of the time, and most nurses are exceptionally skilled and conscientious practitioners, as we have seen. However, unfortunately, this is not the reality 100% of the time and it is important to acknowledge that not all nurses succeed in achieving this goal, as standards of practice vary between different practitioners. In the UK in 2017–18, there were 5,509 new concerns about nurses' fitness to practise raised with the NMC; this equated to about 8 referrals for every 1,000 registrants (NMC 2018) and highlighted significant issues relating to these nurses' 'fitness to practise'.

Every nurse is required to be 'fit to practise' and this means having the skills, knowledge, health and character to do their job safely and effectively. Examples of 'fitness to practise' issues raised in the UK with the NMC are highlighted in Box 6.3.

Box 6.3 Examples of fitness to practise issues raised with the NMC (2018)

- Misconduct (including clinical misconduct) – behaviour that falls short of what is expected of a nurse
- Lack of competence – a lack of knowledge, skill or judgement so that a nurse is incapable of safe and effective practice
- Criminal convictions
- Serious ill health
- Not having the necessary knowledge of the English language.

A nurse's performance will usually have been a cause of concern for some time before a complaint or referral to the relevant professional body is made. Clearly, the performance of all nurses should be monitored locally and causes for concern managed effectively in the local setting so that patients are not put at risk and nurses are supported in improving their performance. This is not just the responsibility of leaders and managers, but of all members of the health professions.

The reasons for poor performance are complex. When nurses make mistakes, for example, it is not usually because they were reckless or lacked skills, but often because the systems in healthcare organisations are not effective in preventing errors or the system rules were not followed for some reason. Organisational and managerial factors can have a stronger influence on errors than the characteristics or behaviour of an individual nurse (Traynor *et al.* 2014). Poor performance can be focused on an individual nurse but may also be a feature of a whole nursing team. An overview of factors leading to poor performance/poor practice in nursing is provided in Box 6.4.

Box 6.4 Factors that can lead to poor performance/poor practice (DeLucia, Ott & Palmieri 2009)

Cognitive factors
- Interruptions – temporarily stopping a task (e.g. medication administration) to perform another task
- Thought processes and decision-making
- Communication processes (see Chapter 4) – including nurse to nurse/health professional, nurse to patient/carer and handovers and care records.

Physical
- Environment – e.g. noise and lighting, layout of patient environment and workspace
- Physical work being carried out
- Nurse's health and well-being – including musculoskeletal disorders related to manual handling tasks.

Organisational
- Working hours – length and time of shifts, number of hours worked per week, etc.
- Staffing resources – staff numbers and staff competencies and skills
- Workload – amount of work to be done in time available
- Stress
- Leadership.

Some practitioners consistently fail to meet standards and some nurses fail in this some of the time because of specific circumstances. For example, short- or long-term health problems or personal circumstances may temporarily affect performance. The Code (NMC 2015, item 8.7, p.11) advises that nurses should: *'be supportive of colleagues who are encountering health or performance problems. However, this support must never compromise or be at the expense of patient or public safety'*. In the UK, the general public or other health professionals can refer a registered nurse to the NMC if they have concerns about their 'fitness to practise' and the NMC is legally bound to investigate all referrals. A nurse or midwife is considered fit to practise when they: *'...have the skills, knowledge, health and character to do their job safely and effectively'* (NMC 2015).

Learning activity 6.3 Developing insight into your own performance

1. Think hard about your own performance as a nurse, in terms of ensuring that patients are safe and that they receive a high standard of care. Over your career so far, have you received constructive feedback aimed at helping you to improve your performance?
2. Thinking back to a time when you received feedback. How did you feel? How did you react and what did you do?

1. Think hard about your own performance as a nurse, in terms of ensuring that patients are safe and that they receive a high standard of care. Over your career so far, have you received constructive feedback aimed at helping you to improve your performance?
2. Thinking back to a time when you received feedback. How did you feel? How did you react and what did you do?
3. Think about the nursing colleagues you work with now and have worked alongside in the past. Can you identify colleagues whose nursing performance you feel is below the standard the public should expect?
4. What do you believe your individual role to have been in highlighting this performance to your colleague and supporting them in making improvements? It is quite common for nurses to simply ignore the questionable performance of others – so if you did that, be honest with yourself.
5. Think about someone you are currently working alongside. What might be the best way to support them now or help them to improve their performance in the future?

Measuring and evaluating nursing performance can be a useful way to gauge the quality of nursing care provided by individual nurses and across nursing teams. Methods for measuring performance tend to include several main approaches (DeLucia, Ott & Palmieri 2009):

- Competencies (individual) – effective application of knowledge, judgement and skills
- Nursing sensitive quality/performance indicators (individual/team) – measures of the impact that nursing care has on patient outcomes and satisfaction
- Individual performance review – often annually through a process laid down by the nurse's employer and involving discussion with a line manager or clinical supervisor
- Peer review – an evaluation of an individual's work performance made by their peers.

Learning activity 6.4 Tackling poor practice

Sam is a newly qualified staff nurse in the sixth week of her first job after qualifying – working in a clinical area she did not experience as a student. Over the last few weeks, she has become increasingly concerned about the practice of another, more experienced, qualified nurse. Some of the other staff talk about this nurse in the staff rest room – they clearly know that the practice of this individual has been a concern for some time and Sam feels that they are fully aware of the situation but have chosen not to act. Sam does not wish to collude with this silence because she feels that this nurse's practice negatively affects quality of care and patient safety.

Sam considers and makes a list of her options:

1. She could approach the member of staff in question and discuss her concerns with them in the spirit of support
2. She could speak to the ward manager about her concerns

3. She could speak to a more senior staff nurse whom she trusts, and seek her advice

4. She could talk it through with some of her colleagues to gain their support in tackling the problem

5. She could telephone the professional body to seek the advice of someone there about her concerns.

Think about each of these approaches.

- What are the possible implications and outcomes for each one?
- Which do you think has the best chance of success?
- How might each one impact on the nurse whom Sam is concerned about?
- What impact might each approach have on the wider nursing and healthcare team?
- What are the implications for Sam?
- Might it be useful to combine two or more of these options?

In the UK, the NMC revalidation process requires every nurse and midwife to regularly demonstrate that they practise safely and meet the standards set out in the *Code* (NMC 2015) and this can be used as an opportunity to tackle poor performance. However, nurses can be reluctant to report their concerns about other members of the healthcare team, often because of fear of victimisation and also because it takes courage to act on such concerns. Moral courage is required: the ability to rise above fear and act according to the values and beliefs of great nursing, overcoming pressure to conform or collude with poor practice. Doing the right thing means thinking carefully about the right approach (Bickhoff, Sinclair & Levett-Jones 2017). Tackling and managing poor practice is a difficult task and, for the novice leader, this will require support from a more senior leader who can help the member of staff to recognise and tackle their competence and fitness to practise through education, learning, coaching and supervision. Treating colleagues with dignity and respect is central to this process.

Conclusion

An individual and team culture of continuous learning is an essential aspect of great nursing. A learning and development culture is likely to be most effective when it is supported by an effective leadership model and every team member is involved. Willingness and skill in supporting others in their learning clearly reflects nursing values. The qualities of a great coach and leader are linked with the 'head, heart and hand' approach discussed throughout this book and reflect the values discussed in Chapter 2. Poor practice is a feature of individuals and teams who lack attention to nursing values and professionalism. A team approach to supporting those whose practice needs improvement is likely to be most effective.

The key points from this chapter can best be summarised in six steps essential for all great nurses wishing to support and influence others – see Box 6.5.

Box 6.5 Steps for great nurses wishing to support and influence others

1. **Share knowledge and skills with others in a culture of collaborative learning.**
2. **Facilitate the learning and development of others using coaching skills linked to the core values of nursing.**
3. **Use transformational leadership skills to support others in becoming great nurses.**
4. **Develop insight into your own performance.**
5. **Support those whose practice needs development by being supportive and respectful.**
6. **Be morally courageous in challenging poor practice.**

Recommendations for further study

Barr, J. & Dowding, L. (2019). *Leadership in healthcare*. 4th edn. London: Sage.

NMC (2019). *Concerns about nurses, midwives or nursing associates*. https://www.nmc.org.uk/concerns-nurses-midwives/ (last accessed 24.1.2020).

Wiggens, L. & Heathershaw, R. (2013). *Mentorship and clinical supervision skills in healthcare*. Andover: CENAGE Learning.

References

Bass, B.M. (1998). *Leadership and performance beyond expectation*. New York: The Free Press.

Bickhoff, L., Sinclair, P. & Levett-Jones, T. (2017). Moral courage in undergraduate nursing students: A literature review. *Collegian*. **24**(1), 71–83.

Bradshaw, A. (2001). *The nurse apprentice: 1860–977*. London: Routledge.

Collins, A., Brown, J.S., & Newman, S.E. (1989). 'Cognitive apprenticeship: Teaching the crafts of reading, writing, and mathematics' in: L.B. Resnick (ed.) *Knowing, learning, and instruction: Essays in honour of Robert Glaser*. pp. 453–94. Hillsdale, New Jersey: Lawrence Erlbaum Associates.

Cummins, A. (2009). Clinical supervision: The way forward? A review of the literature. *Nurse Education in Practice*. **9**(3), 215–20,

DeLucia, P., Ott, T. & Palmieri, P. (2009). Performance in nursing. *Reviews of Human Factors and Ergonomics*. **5**(1), 1–40. https://doi.org/10.1518/155723409X448008 (last accessed 24.1.2020).

Drey, N., Gould, D. & Allan, T. (2009). The relationship between continuing professional education and commitment to nursing. *Nurse Education Today*. **29**(7), 740–45.

Duff, B. (2013). Creating a culture of safety by coaching clinicians to competence. *Nurse Education Today*. **33**(10), 1108–11.

Echeverria, I.L., Patterson, B.J. & Krouse, A. (2017). Predictors of transformational leadership of nurse managers. *Journal of Nursing Management*. **25**, 167–75.

Fahlberg, B. & Toomey, R. (2016). Servant leadership: a model for emerging nurse leaders. *Nursing*. **46**(10), 49–52.

Frankel, A. (2011). What leadership styles should senior nurses develop? *Nursing Times*. **104**(35), 23–24. https://www.nursingtimes.net/clinical-archive/leadership/what-leadership-styles-should-senior-nurses-develop-29-08-2008/ (last accessed 24.1.2020).

Huybrecht, S., Loeckx, W., Quaeyhaegens, Y., De Tobel, D. & Mistiaen, W. (2011). Mentoring in nursing education: Perceived characteristics of mentors and the consequences of mentorship. *Nurse Education Today*. **31**(3), 274–78.

Kelton, M.F. (2014). Clinical coaching – An innovative role to improve marginal nursing students' clinical practice. *Nurse Education in Practice.* **14**(6), 709–13.

The King's Fund (2015). *Leadership and Leadership Development in Healthcare.* https://www.kingsfund.org.uk/sites/default/files/field/field_publication_file/leadership-leadership-development-health-care-feb-2015.pdf (last accessed 24.1.2020).

Kowalski, K. & Casper, C. (2007). The coaching process: An effective tool for professional development. *Nursing Administration Quarterly.* **31**(2), 171–79.

Lee, N.-J. (2011). An evaluation of CPD learning and impact upon positive practice change. *Nurse Education Today.* **31**(4), 390–95

Manley, K., Martin, A., Jackson, C. & Wright, T. (2018). A realist synthesis of effective continuing professional development (CPD): A case study of healthcare practitioners' CPD. *Nurse Education Today.* **69**, 134–41,

Mossiani, G., Bagnasco, A. & Sasso, L. (2017). How staff nurses perceive the impact of nurse managers leadership style in terms of job satisfaction: a mixed methods study. *Journal of Nursing Management.* **25**, 119–28.

Nursing and Midwifery Council (NMC) (2015). *The Code: Professional standards of practice and behaviour for nurses, midwives and nursing associates.* https://www.nmc.org.uk/globalassets/sitedocuments/nmc-publications/nmc-code.pdf (last accessed 24.1.2020).

Nursing and Midwifery Council (NMC) (2018). *Annual Fitness to Practise Report 2017–2018.* https://www.nmc.org.uk/globalassets/sitedocuments/annual_reports_and_accounts/ftpannualreports/annual-fitness-to-practise-report-2017-2018-web.pdf (last accessed 24.1.2020).

Spence Laschinger, H.K., Wong, C.A., Grau, A.L., Read, E.A. & Stam, L.M.P. (2011). The influence of leadership practices and empowerment on Canadian nurse manager outcomes. *Journal of Nursing Management.* **20**, 877–88.

Stalmeijer, R., Dolmans, D., Wolfhagen, I. & Scherpbier, A. (2009). Cognitive apprenticeship in clinical practice: can it stimulate learning in the opinion of students. *Advances in Health Science Education.* **14**, 535–46.

Tee, S., Jowett, R. & Bechelet-Carter, C. (2009). Evaluation study to ascertain the impact of the clinical academic coaching role for enhancing student learning experience within a clinical masters education programme. *Nurse Education in Practice.* **9**(6) 377–82.

Traynor, M., Stone, K., Cook, H., Gould, D. & Maben, J. (2014). Disciplinary processes and the management of poor performance among UK nurses: bad apple or systemic failure? A scoping study. *Nursing Inquiry.* **21**(1), 51–58. https://doi.org/10.1111/nin.12025 (last accessed 24.1.2020).

Whitmore, J. (2017). *Coaching for performance. Principles and practice of coaching and leadership.* 5th edn. London: Nicholas Brealey.

Yukl, G. (2013). *Leadership in organizations.* Boston: Pearson. https://www.academia.edu/35120132/Yukl_Gary._Leadership_in_Organizations (last accessed 24.1.2020).

Chapter 7

Patient perceptions of great nursing care

Introduction

One of the key principles which forms the central core of best practice in nursing is the use of 'hand, heart and head' to meet the wide range of patient needs that great nurses are likely to encounter. So far, this book has focused on what nurses, believe to be best practice in providing this care. However, it is important to recognise that those who use nursing services may not always feel the same way. In this chapter, the focus will move away from nurse-centred views of excellence to a consideration of what patients actually want, and how they perceive the quality of care they are receiving.

What do patients want from nurses?

It is important to recognise that it is not always easy to find out what patients want from nursing care. As discussed throughout this book, nurses work with a wide range of people, in many different places and environments, and all these people have varying needs and may be from very different cultures and backgrounds. As patients encompass many different types of people and personalities, they are likely to hold widely varying views about what constitutes great nursing care. Requirements for great nursing can also change according to the situation. For example, what might constitute great nursing care in an acute emergency situation may not be appropriate when caring for someone who is chronically ill or at the end of their life. This diversity makes the nurse's role extremely complex. Clearly, the care that satisfies one patient's needs may not satisfy the needs of another.

Consequently, it has become much easier to focus on what can be best described as poor or inadequate nursing practice, rather than highlighting nursing care which is considered excellent (see Chapter 6, Box 6.3). This may simply be because a lack of great nursing care is easier to describe, whereas the presence of excellent nursing care is more likely to go unrecognised because it is the usual, normative expectation. However, this does not mean that patient and carer dissatisfaction should be ignored or that their dissatisfaction has no good cause. One of the key characteristics of a great nurse is their ongoing ability to listen, learn and improve as well as to challenge poor practice.

In the UK, the NMC (2018) provides a range of information specifically designed to inform members of the public about what they can expect from nursing care. The NMC acknowledges that, at the heart of care, patients 'want to feel safe, looked after and listened to'.

The importance of listening to patient views and responding to feedback has long been recognised, with many initiatives all over the world being designed to understand the patient experience of nursing care and improve public involvement and patient empowerment (Brookes & Baker 2017). Large-scale examples include the *World Health Report* (WHO 2000) and the introduction, in 2001, of the NHS annual inpatient survey. However, despite these well-supported initiatives, there remains a gap between what patients want from nursing care and what they actually experience. This is best demonstrated in several reports detailing patients' and carers' dissatisfaction with the care they have received.

In the UK, there have been several widely reported cases of poor nursing care (Department of Health 2012, Francis 2013) (see Chapter 1, Box 1.4). Although it is generally hoped that these are isolated examples of poor practice (Aiken *et al.* 2018), lack of patient satisfaction with nursing care is never far from the headlines (*Guardian* 2017). Much of this has been associated with what is termed 'missed care' where nurses have been too busy to attend fully to some patients' needs. In this situation, comforting actions are minimal, conversations are rushed and medications are given at the wrong time, for example. As well as dissatisfaction, this can lead to an erosion of patient confidence not only in the nurse but in the whole healthcare environment. There is also some emerging research evidence linking levels of satisfaction with nursing care directly to staffing levels: higher nursing staffing levels lead to improved levels of patient satisfaction; and lower staffing levels lead to an increased risk of patient mortality (for more on this, see Siegrist 2013 and Aiken *et al.* 2018).

It's important to recognise that when information about levels of satisfaction is collected, this is generally considered to be 'personal opinion'. The issues patients tend to comment on are unlikely to focus on the technical aspects of care (the 'hand and head'); it's much more common for patients to mention human caring issues, identified as those of 'the heart'. This is clearly illustrated in the findings of Brookes and Baker (2017) who reviewed 228,113 items of online patient feedback from the NHS Choices website, and found that issue of technical competence accounted for only 10% of the feedback items. Box 7.1 lists the top eight reasons for patients reporting positive satisfaction.

Box 7.1 Top eight reasons for positive patient satisfaction

1. Good interpersonal skills
2. Good communication skills
3. Technically competent
4. Patient-centred
5. Efficient
6. Hard-working
7. Clean facilities
8. Good food.

(Taken from: Brookes and Baker 2017)

Interestingly, when looking at the top eight reasons for patients reporting negative levels of satisfaction (Box 7.2), many of the same issues were raised.

Box 7.2 Top eight reasons for treatment being negatively evaluated

1. Poor interpersonal skills
2. Lack of appointment availability
3. Technically incompetent
4. Poor communication skills
5. Lack of aftercare
6. Unclean facilities
7. Difficulty accessing test results
8. Lack of seating and space in waiting areas.
(Taken from: Brookes and Baker 2017)

Clearly, nurses are not responsible for all the issues which Brookes and Baker identify as causes of patient dissatisfaction, and their findings are expressed using a broad-brush approach, which fails to differentiate between different healthcare professionals and different healthcare settings. However, the size of their study and the high levels of consistency between their findings and those of others (Palese *et al.* 2011, Siegrist 2013) gives it some value when trying to identify more clearly what patients want from great nurses and how they perceive the care they receive.

Interpersonal skills appear to be central to the patient experience; and communication is clearly a powerful modifying factor in meeting patient needs (as discussed in Chapter 4). Good communication leads to improved patient satisfaction, and poor communication leads to the opposite. The need to feel 'listened to' not only affects satisfaction with communication, but also has a major impact on patient's perceptions of personalised individual care, and the 'patient-centeredness' of their own treatment as well as patient safety.

Although these findings may appear daunting, great nurses can take heart from them. It is clear that patient's perceptions of nursing care are straight forward. Patients want four key things:

1. Clear communication – where patients feel listened to
2. Nurses with good interpersonal skills, who treat people with politeness and respect
3. To be considered an individual – with their own unique needs
4. To be treated competently.

The majority of patients already perceive the quality of the care they receive from nurses as very high. Brookes and Baker (2017) report that positive evaluations occurred roughly three times more frequently than negative evaluations, with similar levels of satisfaction also reported internationally (Palese *et al.* 2011, Siegrist 2013). Clearly, there is still some way to go; missed care as a potential result of poor staffing levels remains a serious threat to great nursing practice, but recognising what patients want from nurses can only lead to improvements in practice.

Learning activity 7.1. What do patients want from nurses?

One of the most important things patients want from nurses is to be listened to.

Think about a recent patient care experience where you were meeting with a patient for the first time.

- How did you make that patient feel listened to?
- List the things you did that made the patient feel like you had listened. Now think about your list.
- Are there other things you could have done which would have helped?
- Could you have improved on the things you did? (If you are not sure about this, have a look at some of the ideas in Chapter 4 on effective nursing.)

Think about how you could have used the 'hand, heart and head' approach. List the things you could improve.

- How do you think you can bring about these improvements next time you meet a new patient for the first time?

Working in partnership with patients and families

One way to find out 'what patients want from nurses' is for nurses to work in partnership with them. This idea of working in partnership with patients is a relatively new one; and, for some patients and healthcare professionals, it involves a difficult cultural shift away from a traditional, paternalistic relationship. Historically, the evolution of the medical and nursing professions has emphasised the idea of the healthcare professional 'knowing best'; the patient's role has traditionally been described as 'doing what they are told'. Consequently, the idea of working in a patient-centred way that treats people as equal partners in decision-making can be a difficult concept to integrate into practice.

From the healthcare professional's perspective, the need to work in partnership is now enshrined within professional standards, and this is encompassed in many of the core values of nursing practice discussed in Chapter 2. In the UK, the need to work in partnership with patients is also enshrined in legislation, including the Health and Social Care Act (2008/2014) with regulations requiring nurses to ensure that care is patient-centred and designed to meet individual preferences. The 2015 judgement, which involved the UK Supreme Court (Montgomery v Lanarkshire Health Board), clarifies the rights of patients to full disclosure of all information relevant to their healthcare as active partners in healthcare decisions (Griffith 2016).

The American College of Physicians (2018) (Nickel *et al.* 2018) has also published its own position paper on partnership working, which outlines four key principles which should be used to guide partnership working:

1. Patients and families should be treated with dignity and respect
2. Patients and families should be active partners in all aspects of their care

3. Patients and families should contribute to the development and improvement of healthcare systems

4. Patients and families should be partners in the education of healthcare professionals.

Examples of strategies they suggest for directly improving 1:1 partnership working include:

- Asking patients how they prefer to be addressed
- Using language patients understand
- Listening without interruption
- Mutually agreeing on decision goals
- Promoting patient self-management.

Additionally, linked to principles 3 and 4, there are several suggestions about how partnership working can be extended beyond direct 1:1 patient interactions, towards more strategic levels of work. These include:

- Establishing patient and family councils
- Involving patients and families in reviewing and designing patient education material
- Including patients and families in training events and curriculum design
- Including patients and families in the assessment of healthcare staff.

The benefits of working in partnership with patients are becoming well established; apart from increased patient satisfaction with care received, there is also evidence to suggest that partnership working at the 1:1 level can result in improvements in self-management of health conditions and longer-term improved patient outcomes (NHS Confederation 2016).

In a similar way to the American College of Physicians' principles 3 and 4, partnership working can be extended to the wider community, in the form of public and patient partnership with healthcare providers. In the UK, for instance, the public are involved in the work of the regional Clinical Commissioning Groups (CCGs) who determine the type of health resources needed for a particular area and then commission those resources. There are also Patient Partnership Councils within NHS Trusts.

In addition, partnership working at strategic levels can take a less direct route through the use of activist-directed campaigns. These are generally context-specific, such as the campaign organised by haemophilia patients and their families in response to the global contaminated blood products scandal (the Haemophilia Society) or in response to threatened health service changes or closures (Hands off Our Hospital). Many such campaigns successfully demonstrate the need for change while providing opportunities for people to directly express their own healthcare needs and preferences.

Working in partnership with patients and their carers is a positive step towards finding out what expectations of great nursing care look like, but it is important to remember that patients and their carers are not necessarily united in their views. For example, a three-month study by Mukhopadhyay *et al.* (2016) found multiple incidences of clear differences in satisfaction with care received between patients and their family members during admission to an intensive care unit. As Mukhopadhyay (2016) suggests, this divergence in views makes it even more difficult for the nurse to provide excellent care which meets the needs and expectations of both the family/carers and the patient.

Another rarely considered question is whether or not healthcare workers and patients actually *want* to work in partnership? Most regulatory and professional guidance never questions the assumptions underlying the view that partnership working is best practice, and few healthcare professionals or regulators openly suggest that partnership working may not always be appropriate.

Nurses recognise that care is both person- and situation-specific; and, in some situations and for some individuals, it is not always possible to work in partnership. There are patients who may simply be too ill to understand the information given and make informed decisions about their own care. Likewise, some patients with severe mental ill health, those who are not conscious, or young children or those with intellectual disabilities may not be capable of working in partnership in a full or meaningful way. Furthermore, some patients may consciously reject the idea of patient partnership because they quite simply 'don't want to know'.

In these instances, the commonly accepted practice is for healthcare professionals to work in partnership with the patient's family or close friends. Again, however, this is not always satisfactory as families do not necessarily know a patient's wishes, they may never have been in this situation before and it may be something they have never discussed. Families and carers may also be suffering from stress and anxiety, which can impact on their own decision-making abilities. These problems can be further compounded by the uncertain relationship between the patient and their family and friends, of which healthcare professionals can never be certain. Are the family members close to the patient? Are they well intentioned? Finally, family members themselves may not necessarily agree on what they believe a patient's preferences to be, leaving the nurse to deal with competing and potentially opposing care decisions.

Although most healthcare professionals are open to the positive aspects of working in partnership with patients, they are also aware of the potential complexities and difficulties. These problems may come to the fore when patients make decisions that are contrary to the professional's understanding of what constitutes best practice, such as patients who decide to use alternative therapies instead of following conventional treatment pathways or those who continue with risky health behaviours despite medical advice. A notable example is the growing issue of parents deciding to refuse childhood vaccinations (contrary to healthcare professionals' advice, and based on erroneous information), which has led to the resurgence of measles, mumps and rubella, which are potentially very serious diseases. This problem has become so widespread that the World Health Organisation has listed vaccine hesitancy as one of its top ten threats to global health (WHO 2019).

Working in partnership with patients and families is complex and multifaceted but, as great nurses already know, working with people in frequently stressful situations is never easy or straightforward. Most importantly, the fact that partnership working is not easy does not mean it is impossible or should be dismissed or neglected. Great nurses are constantly learning; and learning from what patients, their families and carers think about their care can provide vital information and lead to direct improvements in all aspects of healthcare practice.

Learning activity 7.2 Partnership

Think about where you work now.

- How open is your clinical practice area to working in partnership with patients?
- Rate your clinical area's approach to partnership working on a scale of 1–10 (1 means it's not happening at all and 10 means you are doing all the right things).
- Next time you get a chance, ask your colleagues at work the same question (maybe during a coffee break).
- When you have been able to ask a few people, compare scores and share your findings with the staff you have asked and your clinical manager.
- If you are doing well, a pat on the back is in order, but most areas have some room for improvement and you can use this as a starting point for conversations about how to move positive partnership working a little further forward.

Seeking and responding to patient feedback

Although working in partnership is not always easy or straightforward, partnership working has a positive contribution to make towards the development of best nursing care. If great nurses need to work in partnership to identify what patients perceive as great nursing care, the next question is how they are going to do this.

Siegrist (2013) highlights several common misconceptions amongst healthcare professionals, which can have a negative impact on both seeking and responding to patient feedback. These can be summarised as:

- Few patients complete satisfaction surveys
- Patients who do complete satisfaction surveys are generally unhappy
- Additional comments are only from unhappy patients
- Patient satisfaction doesn't measure the quality of care and, instead, is about popularity
- Patient satisfaction can be improved by making cosmetic changes to the healthcare environment
- Patient satisfaction cannot be improved quickly.

Although some of these misconceptions about patient satisfaction are still prevalent, Siegrist (2013) presents clear evidence of a link between high levels of patient satisfaction and higher-quality patient care, with lower mortality rates, improved patient safety and more clinically effective care in areas with higher levels of patient satisfaction. This finding is strongly supported by the subsequent work of Doyle, Lennox and Bell (2013), while a later study by Aiken *et al.* (2018) clearly identifies that patient satisfaction scores can be directly related to ward staffing levels, with lower staffing levels resulting in lower patient satisfaction.

Clearly, there are strong arguments for seeing patient feedback as beneficial to both monitoring and improving care, and it is well worth taking time to gather information on patient's views and perceptions of the care they receive. As Doyle, Lennox and Bell (2013) assert, patient satisfaction cannot be dismissed as either 'too subjective' or 'mood orientated' and, instead, has considerable value as a clear indicator of standards of clinical practice.

From this it would appear obvious that, at the 1:1 level, a great nurse could simply ask a patient or their family what they think about the care they have received. However, there is evidence that few nurses openly ask individual patients direct questions about their satisfaction with care. In an international study across four countries, Topaz *et al.* (2016) found that only 12% of nurses asked this question directly, and this figure dropped to 7.4% in the UK. The reasons for these low rates are unclear, given that most nurses in the Topaz study (91.6%) felt that talking about patient satisfaction was an important issue.

However, asking patients and families directly about the care they are receiving within a healthcare setting may not always be the best way forward. Asking direct questions of individuals currently undergoing treatment or nursing care raises a number of ethical issues, including vulnerability, coercion, peer pressure and the possibility that patients may simply say what they think the nurse wants to hear because of the intensely dependent nature of the nurse-patient relationship at that time (Economic and Social Research Council 2019). Although asking about patient satisfaction is not necessarily considered 'research', it may involve many of the same ethical issues.

In an attempt to avoid some of these potential ethical issues, other approaches to seeking information about patients' perceptions of care have been adopted. For instance, patients and carers have been asked about their experiences of care after the care episode has taken place and they are no longer in a directly dependent situation. This request for feedback can also take several different forms, including paper-based questionnaires, paper-based suggestion boxes, online surveys, mobile phone-based text messaging rating scales, and push-button 'traffic light' scoring systems in key locations in healthcare settings. Many of these are completely anonymous at source, and where this is not the case (such as text messaging and online surveys), data is normally anonymised prior to being circulated and published (Mahmud 2012).

In the UK, the NHS supports two different approaches to seeking patient feedback: the Friends and Family Test (FFT), and the Patient Advice and Liaison Service (PALS). The NHS FFT was launched in 2013 and offers a straightforward approach to obtaining feedback which is quick, voluntary and anonymous. It asks one simple question: 'how likely are you to recommend our service to friends and family if they need similar care or treatment?' Responses to the question are then ranked from 'extremely likely' to 'extremely unlikely', with an opportunity to leave comments. The NHS PALS offers a complementary service designed to offer confidential advice and support on a range of health-related matters. This includes general health or NHS information, but can also include advice about how to resolve an existing problem, make a complaint or get more involved in the NHS as a layperson/volunteer.

There are also several independent bodies who actively seek and collect feedback, as well as many ways in which individuals can now post comments about their experiences of care, including via social media. Additionally, several patient action groups actively seek to collect patients' views about their healthcare; these are independent of healthcare providers or professional organisations, although some of these groups, such as Patient Opinion, may feed directly into NHS quality processes.

Based on all this evidence, it is increasingly clear that there are now many opportunities for patients and their families to express their views about the healthcare they have received, either privately or publicly, with multiple platforms, forums and methods of providing information. However, this raises further issues. What happens to this feedback? How is it used? And does it make any difference?

Great nurses recognise the importance of continuously learning; and learning from patient feedback is an essential element of maintaining and improving great nursing care. However, many healthcare professionals, including nurses, find it difficult to respond to patient feedback. This is articulated by Sheard, Peacock and Marsh (2018) who, in a UK study exploring ward-based nurses' use of patient feedback, found that many nurses struggled with the diverse nature of the feedback provided, as well as frequently questioning its value and validity.

Information obtained by the NHS from both the Friends and Family Test and PALS is routinely reported in the public domain on a variety of websites, as is information gathered by the CQC and CCGs in the form of publicly accessible online reports. Information from independent sources is normally within the public domain and may also be forwarded to a variety of healthcare provider organisations, including the NHS and CCG.

However, the real purpose of collecting information on patient views and satisfaction is to use it to improve practice and, although these multiple sources may appear beneficial in obtaining clear information about patient perceptions, their sheer variety can often make it difficult to assimilate that information. The complexity of the process can also make it possible to subject the patient feedback to a variety of different interpretations.

At a basic level, many organisations use a simple feedback initiative known as 'You said, we did' to highlight key issues patients may have raised and the responses they have received. This system works well for simple issues (such as improving a catering service or changing opening hours) but it is less effective when dealing with more complex issues (such as patients wanting to be more involved in their own healthcare), which require a multi-faceted approach to arrive at a solution. As a general rule, complex issues generally require complex solutions, not easy answers.

Learning activity 7.3 Feedback

Think about where you work now.

In this chapter we have looked at several ways in which patient feedback can be gathered and where it can be found. It is vital that great nurses are aware of the patient feedback received in their own immediate and local areas, but also more generally.

Please go online and find a relevant patient feedback website (in the UK this could be the CQC, the CCG or the NHS sites) and see what information you can find out about patients' perceptions of care in your area.

- Are patients leaving positive feedback?
- If so, what do they value?
- If they are leaving negative feedback, what issues are they identifying?
- How many of those issues are relevant to your practice area?
- How many of those issues are relevant to nursing care?
- Are they things you need to respond to in your own practice? (NB: Just because they may not mention your practice area directly doesn't mean they aren't relevant.)

Results for NHS Friends and Family test: https://www.nhs.uk/using-the-nhs/about-the-nhs/friends-and-family-test-fft/

CQC inspection reports: https://www.cqc.org.uk/publications

CCG reports and publications: https://www.england.nhs.uk/publication/

Conclusion

Patient perceptions of what great nursing care looks like can vary considerably. Just as individuals differ, views on care can be equally diverse. Partnership working is generally considered to be a positive approach to bridging the potential gap between what patients expect from care, and what nurses and other healthcare professionals think they are delivering. Partnership working is not perfect, from the point of view of patients and families or healthcare professionals, and it doesn't always work as well as it should. Nevertheless, the clear benefits of the partnership approach make it an essential component of great nursing practice.

Patient feedback is also vital to bridge this gap, and there is a clear link between patient satisfaction and standards of practice. Listening to what patients have to say, by whatever means, and then actively responding to their feedback, is also integral to the lifelong learning that lies at the heart of effective patient-focused practice.

Great nurses need to be able to respond to the potentially complex and difficult issues patients may raise, in order to close the gap between what patients want and the care they actually receive. This requires all the skills of 'hand, heart and head', as well as adherence to core values, clear communication and openness to lifelong learning. Great nurses also need to be able to support others in order to deliver effective and responsive partnership working that meets actual needs, clearly voiced by patients.

The key points from this chapter can best be summarised in five steps that are essential for all great nurses wishing to assimilate and act on patient perceptions – see Box 7.3.

Box 7.3 Being a great nurse – patient perceptions

1. Ensure patients feel actively listened to.
2. Always work in partnership with patients whenever possible.

3. Actively seek patient feedback, both good and bad.

4. Remain open to continuous learning from patient feedback.

5. Integrate actions as a direct result of feedback into patient care.

References

Aiken, L.H., Sloane, D.M., Ball, J., Bruyneel, L., Rafferty, A.M. & Griffiths, P. (2018). Patient satisfaction with hospital care and nurses in England: an observational study. *BMJ Open.* https://bmjopen.bmj.com/content/bmjopen/8/1/e019189.full.pdf (last accessed 28.1.2020).

Brookes, G. & Baker, P. (2017). What does patient feedback reveal about the NHS? A mixed methods study of comments posted to the NHS choices online service. *BMJ Open.* https://bmjopen.bmj.com/content/bmjopen/7/4/e013821.full.pdf (last accessed 28.1.2020).

Department of Health (DH) (2012). *Transforming Care: a national response to Winterbourne View Hospital, Department of Health Review, Final Report.* https://www.gov.uk/government/uploads/system/uploads/attachment_data/file/213215/final-report.pdf (last accessed 28.1.2020).

Doyle, C., Lennox, L. & Bell, D. (2013). A systematic review of evidence on the links between patient experience and clinical safety and effectiveness. *BMJ Open.* 3(1). https://bmjopen.bmj.com/content/3/1/e001570 (last accessed 28.1.2020).

Economic and Social Research Council (2019). *Research with potentially vulnerable people.* https://esrc.ukri.org/funding/guidance-for-applicants/research-ethics/frequently-raised-topics/research-with-potentially-vulnerable-people/ (last accessed 28.1.2020).

Francis, R. (2013). *The Midstaffordshire NHS Foundation Trust Public Inquiry.* http://webarchive.nationalarchives.gov.uk/20150407084003/http://www.midstaffspublicinquiry.com/ (last accessed 28.1.2020).

Guardian (2017). *NHS Nurses are too busy to care for patients properly.* https://www.theguardian.com/society/2017/sep/29/nhs-nurses-are-too-busy-to-care-for-patients-properly-research-shows (last accessed 28.1.2020).

Griffith, R. (2016). The changing nature of the nurse-patient partnership. *British Journal of Neuroscience Nursing.* 12(5), 246–47.

Mahmud, T. (2012). *Better patient feedback, better healthcare.* Keswick: M&K Update Ltd.

Mukhopadhyay, A., Son, G., Sim, P.Z., Ting, K.C., Yoo, J.K.S., Want, Q.L., Mascuri, R.B.H.M., Ong, V.H.L., Phua, J. & Kowitlawakul, Y. (2016). Satisfaction domains differ between the patient and their family in adult intensive care units. *Biomedical Research International.* https://doi.org/10.1155/2016/9025643 (last accessed 28.1.2020).

NHS Confederation (2016). *Public and patient partnership. How they can address the inequality and finance gap in healthcare.* https://www.nhsconfed.org/-/media/Confederation/Files/Publications/Documents/Public-and-patient-partnerships-WEB.pdf (last accessed 28.1.2020).

Nickel, W.K., Weinberger, S.E. & Guze, P.A. (2018). Principles of patient and family partnership in care: an American College of Physicians Position Paper. *Annals of Internal Medicine.* **169**(11), 796–98.

Nursing and Midwifery Council (NMC) (2018). *Good nursing and midwifery care.* https://www.nmc.org.uk/globalassets/sitedocuments/nmc-publications/nmc-code-patient-public-leaflet.pdf (last accessed 28.1.2020).

Palese, A., Tomietto, M., Suhonen, R., Efstathiou, G., Tsangari, H., Merkouris, A., Jarosova, D., Leino-Kilp, H., Patiraki, E., Karlou, C., Balogh, Z. & Papastavrou, E. (2011). Surgical patient satisfaction as an outcome of nursing caring behaviours: a descriptive and correlational study of six European countries. *Journal of Nursing Scholarship.* **43** (4), 341–50.

Sheard, L., Peacock, R. & Marsh, C. (2018). What's the problem with patient experience feedback? A macro and micro understanding based on findings from a three site UK qualitative study. *Health Expectations.* **22**, 46–53.

Siegrist, R.B. (2013). History of medicine. Patient satisfaction; history, myths and misperceptions. *American Medical Association Journal of Ethics.* **15**(11), 982–87.

Topaz, M., Lisby, M., Morrison, C.P.R.C., Levtzion-Korach, O., Hockey, P.M., Salzberg, C.A., Efrati, N., Lipsitz, S., Bates, D.W. & Rozenblum, R. (2016). Nurse's perspectives on patient satisfaction and expectations: an international cross-sectional multicentre study with implications for evidence-based practice. *Worldviews on Evidence-Based Nursing.* **13**(3), 185–96.

World Health Organization (2019). *Ten threats to global health in 2019.* https://www.who.int/emergencies/ten-threats-to-global-health-in-2019 (last accessed 28.1.2020).

World Health Organization (WHO) (2000). *The world health report 2000.* http://apps.who.int/gb/archive/pdf_files/WHA53/ea4.pdf (last accessed 28.1.2020).

Sources of further information

For more information about Clinical Commissioning Groups please look at:
https://www.england.nhs.uk/ccgs/ (last accessed 29.1.2020).

For more information about the Care Quality Commission please look at:
https://www.cqc.org.uk/ (last accessed 29.1.2020).

For more information about the Haemophilia Society and the contaminated blood products campaign please look at:
https://haemophilia.org.uk/support/day-day-living/patient-support/contaminated-blood/history-contaminated-blood/ (last accessed 29.1.2020).

For an example of hospital closure campaign groups, please look at:
Huddersfield Royal Infirmary, Hands off our Hospital.
https://officialhandsoffhri.org/ (last accessed 29.1.2020).

For further information on leaving feedback, please look at:
Care Opinion https://www.careopinion.org.uk/ (last accessed 29.1.2020).
NHS Friends and Family Test (NHS FFT) https://www.nhs.uk/using-the-nhs/about-the-nhs/friends-and-family-test-fft/ (last accessed 29.1.2020).
Patient Advice and Liaison Service (PALS) https://www.nhs.uk/common-health-questions/nhs-services-and-treatments/what-is-pals-patient-advice-and-liaison-service/ (last accessed 29.1.2020).

Chapter 8

Embracing the future of nursing

Introduction

Healthcare moves forward at an alarming pace as the demands of populations develop, and the social, cultural, technological and political influences alter. Over the years, nurses have embraced change and development; never more so than in the last few decades, in which there have been many exciting and challenging developments in the way nursing has advanced. This means that every nurse sees changes in the way care is delivered, and led, in the course of their careers.

In wealthier nations, political influences lead to a demand for more affordable and sustainable healthcare provision. In less affluent nations, providing healthcare at all can be a major challenge. Even in wealthier parts of the world, healthcare budgets have never been more tightly controlled, as governments attempt to curb the rising costs of providing medical care. As the world is more closely linked than ever before, global changes have an increasing impact on the healthcare needs that nurses aim to meet. Global warming is likely to affect everyone, bringing major health implications, both directly and indirectly linked to environmental changes. The world population is changing, with declining birth rates in higher income countries being counter-balanced by increased life expectancy, tipping the overall population towards the older end of the spectrum. We are also facing the growth of man-made health threats, such as antimicrobial resistance (the ability of microorganisms to prevent antibiotics and other antimicrobials from working against them) and air pollution.

A humane and ethical society needs nurses to care for those who are vulnerable and in need. However, modern economics and the changing nature of healthcare requirements means that care-givers, and the systems in which they work, have never been under greater pressure to do more, with ever-shrinking resources.

Having a view of the future is helpful to prepare nurses for challenges that will arise as their careers progress; it also helps ensure that nurses remain effective as conditions change and develop. This chapter provides an overview of some of the challenges and opportunities that will confront nurses in the coming decades, as healthcare, and nursing, develop and change.

Healthcare and the nursing resource

The global population of people over the age of 60 years is now larger than the number of children under the age of 5 years. People are living longer, but there is an increasing incidence of chronic diseases, which means that the demand for healthcare services is likely to keep rising in the coming decades. Global economic growth, modernisation and urbanisation are encouraging unhealthy lifestyles, creating a rise in chronic ill health. People are living longer because of better healthcare. However, while living conditions improve, lifestyle choices that lead to ill health are still a major issue. As people in wealthier nations are often living longer, with more chronic ill health, they need more healthcare than ever before. Despite medical advances, communicable diseases (such as HIV/AIDS, tuberculosis, malaria, ebola and zika virus) continue to devastate communities and create global fear. Antibiotic-resistant strains of pathogenic organisms and pandemic outbreaks challenge healthcare systems in ways never seen before. Nurses respond to the health needs of people in all settings and throughout their lifespan, so they are central to health promotion, disease prevention, treatment, care and rehabilitation (WHO 2016).

The form of capitalism that currently exists in most of the developed world means that there is pressure to provide healthcare at the lowest possible cost, whilst still making it available to the entire community. In systems where healthcare is privately funded, it often seems that profit is the most important target. As the largest workforce in healthcare systems, nurses are central to the success of healthcare, but also vulnerable to cost-containment measures. Great nurses and nurse leaders are deeply involved in the redesign and development of healthcare systems, making sure that modern capitalism does not compromise on providing high-quality nursing care. In the last few decades, nursing roles have expanded to help health services meet increasing demand for high-quality healthcare.

All over the world, there are shortages of healthcare workers. In the UK, fewer nurses are being trained and more nurses are leaving the profession. As large numbers of experienced nurses retire, and it becomes increasingly challenging to recruit new nurses, the nursing workforce in many developed countries has begun to shrink (NMC 2018).

Nurses make up the largest proportion of the healthcare workforce because they provide the most care across the full 24-hour period. However, as discussed in Chapter 1, the nursing role is very diverse and nurses often have some difficulty in:

- Explaining what they do
- Explaining how and why what they do makes so much difference to individuals and communities
- Acting as advocates for patients whose care is affected negatively by nursing shortages.

Because nursing activity is so complex, identifying its positive impact on patient outcomes can be difficult. However, in the last decade or so, the nursing profession has become better at demonstrating its impact by measuring nurse-sensitive outcomes (Maben *et al.* 2012). Even so, healthcare organisations are under pressure to provide more expensive medical care to more people at lower cost, and this this often places nurses under additional pressure while making them vulnerable to staffing reductions. In the hospital setting, for example, as the length of patient stays is reduced, the care they need is concentrated into a shorter space of time and nurses need to provide that care under greater pressure. This also demands more of nursing values and nurses' ability to constantly give care with the 'head, heart and hand'. Although nurses have adapted to this situation by developing resilience to these stresses (as discussed in Chapter 5), this situation is constantly discussed and debated by nurses and their leaders.

The availability of enough appropriately educated and skilled nurses to provide great care remains a source of anxiety. In a large international study, Aiken *et al.* (2014) demonstrated that an increase in a nurse's workload by one patient (from eight to nine patients per qualified nurse) led to a 7% increase in the likelihood of a surgical inpatient dying within 30 days of surgery. One explanation for this is that the under-resourcing of nursing teams means that there is insufficient capacity for the team to undertake actions to prevent morbidity and mortality. Studies have indicated that this 'missed care' is associated with one or more adverse patient outcomes, including medication errors, urinary tract infections, falls, pressure injuries, critical incidents, and patient readmissions. However, the quality of studies relating to missed care is weak, and the link between missed care and mortality will remain uncertain until further high-quality studies take place (Recio-Saucedo *et al.* 2018).

The solutions to these problems are complex and involve governments, healthcare organisations, organisations representing nurses, and nurses themselves working together. Nurses need to be politically aware and find a voice that enables them to articulate the problems created (for patients and for nurses themselves) by depleted nursing resources.

Learning activity 8.1 Nurse staffing and educational level and patient safety

Access the following important journal article about nurse staffing discussed above:

Aiken, L., Sloane, D. Bryneel, L. *et al.* (2014). Nurse staffing and education and hospital mortality in nine European countries: a retrospective observational study. *Lancet.* **383**(993), 1824–30.

You will be able to access the article through the following link. It is free to download but you may need to register on the system. Alternatively, you could access it through your local health service/ university library:
https://doi.org/10.1016/S0140-6736(13)62631-8

Read the article. It focuses on surgical nursing in a hospital setting but has many things to say about nursing in all specialties and fields.

- As you read the article, reflect on the impact of nurse staffing levels on great nursing.
- Ask yourself how you feel about this and what you think nurses, individually and collectively, should do about it.

Because of the pressures on both healthcare services and on nurses, the nursing profession has had to broaden and develop the roles available to nurses. Registered nurses have always been supported by healthcare assistants or support workers who implement care planned by their registered colleagues. These assistants or support workers are usually staff members with extensive experience, who can provide great care under the supervision of registered practitioners. The global shortage of registered nurses means that new roles have developed to enhance the nursing team and provide career pathways for healthcare assistants and support workers. In the UK, for example, two roles are currently being rolled out (see Box 8.1).

Box 8.1 Nursing Associates and Assistant Practitioners

1. Nursing Associates: Nursing Associates fill a new support role that will sit alongside existing healthcare support workers and registered nurses to deliver hands-on care for patients. They undertake a two-year programme, leading to a foundation degree. A shortened apprenticeship route will also be introduced for qualified Nursing Associates who wish to work towards a degree to obtain registered nurse status with the NMC status.

2. Assistant Practitioners: Assistant Practitioners (also known as Associate Practitioners) can take on more responsibilities than healthcare assistants and are also under the supervision of registered nurses. Many Nursing Associates/Assistant Practitioners will complete a foundation degree in healthcare, involving both study (Head) and supervised practice (Hand). There are plans in place to enable them to use their foundation degree to access a shortened undergraduate degree programme such as a nursing degree.

Royal College of Nursing (2019). *Career paths for Nursing Support Workers.*

https://www.rcn.org.uk/professional-development/your-career/hca/career-paths-for-hcas (last accessed 29.1.2020)

As discussed in Chapter 5, nurses are also being asked to take on a much greater variety of roles, and, in the course of their careers, they may find themselves following a very diverse range of career opportunities. Many of these roles may take the nurse away from direct patient care; they may also involve taking on roles previously undertaken by other healthcare professionals (normally medical staff). Although this expansion of roles has many benefits for the nursing profession and patient care, it can lead to a perception that nurses are sometimes being distracted from what were previously considered core nursing activities.

Ultimately, all these developments mean that registered nurses will work alongside more practitioners with diverse roles, whilst also undertaking a much broader range of roles themselves. Consequently, great nurses will increasingly need to be able to supervise, educate and support those who have chosen these alternative healthcare roles.

Globalisation and transcultural care

Through greater movement of people, goods and ideas across boundaries, globalisation is leading to far-reaching changes in human societies. These changes affect everything, from individual people to vast healthcare systems. Health is no longer confined by national boundaries, and nursing is now being provided for increasingly diverse populations as people move around the world, taking their health problems with them and acquiring new problems in countries where they settle.

Nurses working with patients from diverse backgrounds, with different cultural needs from their own, must be culturally competent in the way they provide care, with a deep appreciation of the lives and values of others through use of both 'the head and the heart'. They must approach the nursing care of individuals with a cultural sensitivity that is truly individualised (Giger 2017), providing transcultural nursing that includes assessments and interventions utilising appropriate and effective communication.

Learning activity 8.2 Cultural competence

Leininger and McFarland (2006) define transcultural nursing care as:

> '…Practice which is focused upon differences and similarities among cultures with respect to human care, health (or well-being), and illness, based upon the people's cultural values, beliefs and practices.'

This means that nurses need relevant culturally specific knowledge and skills to provide great care for everyone, no matter what their background.

- Undertake a web search using terms such as 'transcultural nursing model' and/or 'cultural competence model nursing'.
- Identify three or four named models that relate to great nursing in a transcultural context.
- Choose one of these on which to undertake some further reading, using your web search.
- Think about someone you have cared for recently who had quite different cultural values from your own.
- How might the information you have found help you to give more culturally sensitive care to that person?

The global financial crisis has provided new drivers for nurse migration. Skilled and specialist nurses from countries where nursing jobs are harder to find, and economic conditions are less favourable, are now more likely to migrate. This means that many migrant nurses are leaving economically challenged countries to seek better salaries and working conditions, leaving fewer skilled nurses available to provide care in their countries of origin.

The International Council of Nurses recognises the potential benefits of 'circular' nurse migration, whereby nurses move from one place to another and are replaced as they move by other nurses migrating from elsewhere (ICN 2007). This provides many opportunities for learning and development of multicultural practice. It also promotes self-confidence and the ability to cope with new challenges while embracing different cultures and enables nurses to better meet the needs of those whose culture is different from their own.

Working effectively alongside nurses who undertook their nursing education in other countries leads to greater understanding of their experience. Li, Nie and Lid (2014) highlight some significant negative experiences for migrant nurses, including difficulties in adjusting to new work and social environments, unfamiliarity of place and culture, often being far away from close family members and support networks, challenges of adjusting to new occupational standards, language difficulties and the challenges of forming working relationships. Tregunno *et al.* (2009) quote the following salutary words from migrant nurses themselves to illustrate real experiences of 'being an outsider':

'Most people ... when I talk ... they are like ... they don't understand me ... so I have to talk like three times ... they don't understand me ... I don't understand them ... I have to talk slowly for them to understand ... and they have to talk slowly for me to understand. When I talk with patients, I paraphrase what I said, or in some cases, I may call another nurse and they will explain to the patient' (p. 187–188)

'Some nurses think that because you're an immigrant, you probably are not educated ... [that] you don't know what you are doing ... so they don't have trust in you whenever you're doing something, like when you're doing a procedure on a patient ... or giving medication ...'

'The way the patients talk with the nurses, sometimes they get aggressive ... and some of the patients discriminate ... like when you talk to them ... Oh, don't touch me ... you can hear patients say ... Oh, you're black ... I've had that! They say ... I don't want a black person to touch me. I want a white nurse to give me care ...'

An empathetic understanding of these experiences presents an opportunity for colleagues to welcome practitioners migrating into their workplace. Other team members can make a significant difference, supporting migrant nurses to integrate into their new team by providing supervision, preceptorship, training and education, warmth and friendliness, help with understanding the new environment and compassionate empathetic support.

As well as presenting problems for the individual migrant nurse, migration of a skilled workforce from a developing country to a developed one can create what is known as a 'malicious cycle', on a global level. Although the migrant nurse may be financially better off by working in another country, and this may result in their own family (who are frequently left behind in their original country) also being better provided for, mass migration of skilled nurses results in depletion of their own country's resources. Any financial gain is not fed back into that country's healthcare system, and the depletion of skilled nurses can lead to an inexorable worsening of working conditions and overall nursing care for those left behind (BMJ 2018).

Consequently, globalisation (and the subsequent greater movement of people) can have both positive and negative implications for future nurses and the quality of care patients receive. Decisions made about staff resources and future nurse staffing and education planning should therefore take this much bigger global picture into account.

The environment and sustainability

Climate change is now much discussed; and it is an important consideration in almost everything human beings do. It affects healthcare in many ways – not least due to its impact on public health. The World Health Organization (2018) has identified three major areas in which climate affects the health and wellbeing of communities:

- **Extreme heat** – leading to deaths of, particularly, older people due to cardiac and respiratory events
- **Natural disasters and changing rainfall patterns** – leading to floods and failure of crops and affecting the supply and quality of fresh water

- **Patterns of infection** – climatic conditions affecting insect-, water- and air-borne diseases (such as malaria) which now have longer transmission seasons.

Extreme weather conditions increasingly place people's health at risk and nurses are often at the forefront of dealing with climate disasters such as floods. In rural and less economically advanced areas, climate is having an impact on the production of food. Nurses frequently play an important role in promoting health in extreme climate conditions and in providing care for those affected by extreme events.

Although it is sometimes easy for nurses in the developed world, including the UK, to dismiss many of these climate changes issues as 'happening elsewhere', their impact is likely to be as important, if not quite so dramatic, in the UK. The NHS publishes an annual Heatwave Plan (2019) which is designed to prevent avoidable heat-related deaths during extreme hot weather, initiated by a Heat Health Watch System (NHS 2019), with a parallel Cold Weather Plan (NHS 2018), and it is likely that both of these will be initiated much more frequently in the future.

These global threats mean that it is increasingly vital to manage the resources involved in healthcare carefully – from more judicious use of healthcare equipment and financial resources to making the best use of staffing resources. There is now a growing awareness of the impact of healthcare services on the environment, and healthcare's own contribution to climate change and environmental pollution. For this reason, healthcare services are now focusing on issues such as sustainable waste management, including avoiding the use of single-use items where possible and managing the overall disposal of plastic items from healthcare activity, whilst working to promote the health of those affected by problems created by climate change.

Air pollution is an additional source of concern and an important current topic in the discussion about the impact of the environment on global health. This is a particular problem in cities, where more than half of the world's population now live; and it is expected that by 2030 urban areas will house 60% of the world's population (UN 2016). It is well known that air pollution exacerbates existing asthma, but it is becoming increasingly clear that air pollution is also a primary cause of allergic asthma due to inhalation of particulate matter from vehicle fumes, in particular. There is growing evidence that this is leading to significant health problems and deaths.

Polluted air is also a major contributor to diseases such as chronic obstructive pulmonary disease (COPD), where it is known to result in acute exacerbations and an increased risk of both morbidity and mortality (Jiang, Mei & Feng 2016). Future great nurses will pay a significant role in helping individuals and communities to manage exacerbations of their asthma and COPD, to prevent deaths, but also in educating patients in strategies that will help them to avoid or manage pollution-driven risk factors.

Technology and telehealth

Since the 1990s, technology has been an increasingly important part of healthcare delivery. For several decades, nurses have been accessing information, recording patient assessment, planning care and communicating with other members of their teams using technology. Over the last 30 years, technology has become an essential tool in providing safe and effective care, particularly in the areas of communication, record-keeping, information-gathering and decision-making. It has frequently been demonstrated that, if implemented well, technology can help nurses in their work (Wisner, Lyndon & Chesla 2019).

In the early years of this revolution, many nurses struggled to develop the skills needed to make use of technology in their everyday working lives. Most have risen to the challenge, but they will need to keep themselves abreast of developments as technology continues to advance. Technology is now such an integral part of nursing practice that it is impossible to be a great nurse without having great technology skills as well. These skills are embedded in the NMC's (2019) *Standards of proficiency for registered nurses.*

Learning activity 8.3 Using technology in practice

- Thinking about your last shift or your last direct patient contact, write a list of activities you undertook that involved the use of technology.
- Consider the benefits to patients of the use of technology in some of the situations you have identified.
- Now assess your own competence in using technology in your current nursing activity.
- Identify some gaps in your competence – every nurse has some – and identify some ways in which you might be able to fill those gaps. Do you need more training? How could you access it? What might be the benefit to patients of doing that?
- Do you need to ask someone in your organisation to help you with developing your skills further?
- Do you simply need to spend time practising these skills?

For many nurses, learning to use technology effectively takes time and effort, but it is known to have a positive impact on the nurse's practice and on patient care.

Electronic health records are digital records of patients' health and care. They aim to improve safety by facilitating communication and access to information, reducing errors, supporting decision-making, improving adherence to evidence-based practice guidelines and enabling healthcare professionals to analyse data. See Box 8.2 for an overview of a literature review considering how electronic health records impact on nurses' practice.

Box 8.2 Electronic health records and nurses

Wisner, Lyndon and Chesla (2019) undertook an integrative literature review of studies that had explored the electronic health record's impact on nurses' cognitive work.

The findings of the review were as follows:

'Five themes identified how nurses and other clinicians used the electronic health record and perceived its impact:

1. forming and maintaining an overview of the patient,

2. cognitive work of navigating the electronic health record,

3. use of cognitive tools,

4. forming and maintaining a shared understanding of the patient, and

5. loss of information and professional domain knowledge.

Most studies indicated that forming and maintaining an overview of the patient at both the individual and team level were difficult when using the electronic health record. Navigating the volumes of information was challenging and increased clinicians' cognitive work. Information was perceived to be scattered and fragmented, making it difficult to see the chronology of events and to situate and understand the clinical implications of various data. The template-driven nature of documentation and limitations on narrative notes restricted clinicians' ability to express their clinical reasoning and decipher the reasoning of colleagues. Summary reports and hand over/off tools in the electronic health record proved insufficient as standalone tools to support nurses' work throughout the shift and during hand over/off, causing them to rely on self-made paper forms. Nurses needed tools that facilitated their ability to individualize and contextualize information in order to make it clinically meaningful.'

(Wisner, Lyndon & Chesla 2019, p.74).

Aside from using technology directly focused on the individual patient, telehealth (sometimes known as eHealth) involves the use of communication technology to deliver healthcare remotely from a traditional healthcare facility acting as a hub. Advances in communication technology now allow healthcare practitioners to remotely interact with communities and patients and to monitor their health and wellbeing using computers and telephones. Sometimes this approach is also integrated into traditional care, using the best option for the patient at the time. In the past, this has mainly been used to help people living in remote areas to access healthcare, but it is now becoming an integral part of all healthcare delivery, especially in countries and regions where distances involved are very great.

Nurses are deeply involved in the delivery of telehealth care to individuals and communities where they live and work. This can be particularly helpful in remote communities and for those who find it difficult to travel to hospitals or clinics because of chronic health conditions, disabilities and personal circumstances. It is also seen as economically viable and sustainable because it reduces travel and saves time and cost for both patients and healthcare staff.

Examples of nurses' involvement in telehealth include (van Houwelingen et al. 2016):

- Replacing face-to-face visits with e-visits via the use of video links
- Monitoring health parameters such as blood pressure, blood glucose levels or heart rate via devices for self-measurement
- Monitoring activity in and around the home via activity monitors, e.g. in patients prone to falling

- Responding to personal alarms by patients to let nurses or family members know when help is needed
- Teleconsultation, e.g. providing wound assessment and management advice at a distance.

As well as effectively using technology to support nursing care, many of the skills nurses need for such activities are already a vital part of great nursing. These include the ability to communicate effectively and reduce patient anxiety when using technology with which the patient may be unfamiliar (van Houwelingen *et al.* 2016).

An integral aspect of using technology to support great nursing care is for nurses to be able to use it to access information to support their own nursing practice. In particular, nurses need to be able to find, select, access and understand the best evidence for care. As discussed in Chapters 3 and 4, this not only involves being able to access and evaluate primary research, but also using summaries of evidence, guidelines and protocols for practice. Advanced skills in searching electronically for this material are essential as nursing careers develop.

The technology used in healthcare is likely to advance at an ever faster rate; and it is often hard to grasp the likely impact of these changes on patient care and nursing activity. The most important issues on the horizon are likely to be those involving robotics and artificial intelligence. Replacing nurses with artificially intelligent robots is unlikely in the near future. Nevertheless, it is tempting to consider the idea that a robot might take on some of nursing's more problematic and risky tasks such as patient handling and medication administration. Indeed, robots designed to take on elements of a nurse's role have already been trialled in a number of countries (Nurse.org 2018) .

Learning activity 8.4 Future proofing

- Thinking about the issues raised in this chapter, make a list of three things you think are most central to your own future practice.
- Think about how you could prepare for these in the coming months and years.
- Think about some of the issues considered in Chapter 3 on learning to be a great nurse, and write a plan of action that includes your educational needs.

Conclusion

Nursing practice has never been static. It has always developed to meet the needs of the community and the patients nurses serve. The demand for such developments has never been greater. Despite the many challenges of modern and future healthcare, nurses need to maintain the core values of their profession (discussed in detail in Chapter 2) and make sure they continuously engage with their own professional development (as described in Chapter 3). Great nurses are flexible, responsive and well informed. Great and effective nurses have a range of skills at their disposal, especially the ability to communicate (as discussed throughout this book). Although there are challenges ahead, great nurses will be able to continue using the 'hand, head and heart' to deliver great nursing care, both in the present and the future.

The key points from this chapter can best be summarised in three steps for all great nurses (see Box 8.3 below).

Box 8.3 Three steps to being a great nurse – embracing the future

1. Head: be knowledgeable about social, cultural, environmental, technological and political influences so that you can alter your practice accordingly

2. Heart: ensure that your own future career stays focused on the core values of nursing (as discussed in Chapters 1 and 2), despite influences from outside the profession

3. Hand: maintain your skills and develop new skills to meet the needs of patients in a changing world.

References

Aiken, L., Sloane, D., Bruyneel, L., Van den Heede, K., Griffiths, P., Busse, R., Diomidous, M., Kinnunen, J., Kózka, M., Lesaffre, E., McHugh, M., Moreno-Casbas, M., Rafferty, A., Schwendimann, R., Scott, P., Tishelman, C., van Achterberg, T. & Sermeus, W. (2014). Nurse staffing and education and hospital mortality in nine European countries: a retrospective observational study. *Lancet*. **383**(9931), 1824–30. http://dx.doi.org/10.1016/S0140-6736(13)62631-8 (last accessed 30.1.2020).

British Medical Journal (2018). *Changing how we think about healthcare improvement.* https://www.bmj.com/content/361/bmj.k2014/rr-3 (last accessed 30.1.2020).

Giger, J.N. (2017). *Transcultural nursing. Assessment and intervention.* St Louis: Elsevier.

International Council of Nurses (ICN) (2018). *Policy brief. Nurse Retention.* Geneva: ICN. https://www.icn.ch/sites/default/files/inline-files/ICNM%20Nurse%20retention%20FINAL.pdf Accessed 02.02.2020

Jiang, X.Q., Mei, X.D. & Feng, D. (2016). Air pollution and chronic airway diseases: what should people know and do? *Journal of Thoracic Disease*. **8**(1), E31–40. https://www.ncbi.nlm.nih.gov/pmc/articles/PMC4740163/ (last accessed 30.1.2020).

Li, H., Nie, W. & Lid, J. (2104). The benefits and caveats of international nurse migration. *International Journal of Nursing Sciences*. **1**(3), 314–17.

Leininger, M. & McFarland, M. (2006). *Culture care diversity and universality. A worldwide nursing theory.* 2nd edn. Sudbury: Jones & Bartlett.

Maben, J., Morrow, E., Ball, J., Robert, G. & Griffiths, P. (2012). *High Quality Care Metrics for Nursing.* National Nursing Research Unit, King's College London. https://www.kcl.ac.uk/nmpc/research/nnru/publications/Reports/High-Quality-Care-Metrics-for-Nursing----Nov-2012.pdf (last accessed 30.1.2020).

Nurse.org (2018). *Will These Nurse Robots Take Your Job?* https://nurse.org/articles/nurse-robots-friend-or-foe/ (last accessed 30.1.2020).

Nursing and Midwifery Council (NMC) (2019). *Future Nurse: Standards of proficiency for registered nurses.* https://www.nmc.org.uk/globalassets/sitedocuments/education-standards/future-nurse-proficiencies.pdf (last accessed 30.1.2020).

Recio-Saucedo, A., Dall'Ora, C., Maruotti, A., Ball, J., Briggs, J., Meredith, P., Redfern, O., Kovacs, C., Prytherch, D., Smith, G. & Griffiths, P. (2018). What impact does nursing care left undone have on patient outcomes? Review of the literature. *Journal of Clinical Nursing.* **11–12**, 2248–59.

Tregunno, D., Peters, S., Campbell, H. & Gordon, S. (2009). International nurse migration: U-turn for safe workplace transition. *Nursing Inquiry.* **16**(3), 182–90.

United Nations (UN) (2016). *The world's cities in 2016.* Data booklet. United Nations. New York. https://www.un.org/en/development/desa/population/publications/pdf/urbanization/the_worlds_cities_in_2016_data_booklet.pdf (last accessed 30.1.2020).

van Houwelingen, C., Moerman, A., Ettema, R., Kort, H. & Cate, O. (2016). Competencies required for nursing telehealth activities: A Delphi-study. *Nurse Education Today*. **39**, 50–62.

Wisner, K., Lyndon, A. & Chesla, C. (2019). The electronic health record's impact on nurses' cognitive work: An integrative review. *International Journal of Nursing Studies*. **94**,74–84.

World Health Organization (2016). *Global strategic directions for strengthening nursing and midwifery 2016–2020.* World Health Organization. Geneva. https://www.who.int/hrh/nursing_midwifery/global-strategic-midwifery2016-2020. pdf?ua=1 (last accessed 30.1.2020).

World Health Organization (2018). *Climate Change and Health.* Fact sheet https://www.who.int/news-room/fact-sheets/detail/climate-change-and-health (last accessed 30.1.2020).

Sources of further information

National Health Service (2019). *Heat wave plan for England.* https://assets.publishing.service.gov.uk/government/uploads/system/uploads/attachment_data/file/801539/Heatwave_plan_for_England_2019.pdf (last accessed 30.1.2020).

Nursing and Midwifery Council (NMC) (2018). *The NMC register.* https://www.nmc.org.uk/globalassets/sitedocuments/other-publications/the-nmc-register-2018.pdf (last accessed 30.1.2020).

Honey and Mumford learning styles questionnaire

Learning styles questionnaire

Name: _____

This questionnaire is designed to find out your preferred learning style(s). Over the years you have probably developed learning 'habits' that help you benefit more from some experiences than from others. Since you are probably unaware of this, this questionnaire will help you pinpoint your learning preferences so that you are in a better position to select learning experiences that suit your style and having a greater understanding of those that suit the style of others.

This is an internationally proven tool designed by Peter Honey and Alan Mumford.

There is no time limit to this questionnaire. It will probably take you 10–15 minutes. The accuracy of the results depends on how honest you can be. There are no right or wrong answers.

If you agree more than you disagree with a statement put a tick by it.

If you disagree more than you agree put a cross by it.

Be sure to mark each item with either a tick or cross.

- ☐ 1. I have strong beliefs about what is right and wrong, good and bad.
- ☐ 2. I often act without considering the possible consequences
- ☐ 3. I tend to solve problems using a step-by-step approach
- ☐ 4. I believe that formal procedures and policies restrict people
- ☐ 5. I have a reputation for saying what I think, simply and directly
- ☐ 6. I often find that actions based on feelings are as sound as those based on careful thought and analysis
- ☐ 7. I like the sort of work where I have time for thorough preparation and implementation
- ☐ 8. I regularly question people about their basic assumptions
- ☐ 9. What matters most is whether something works in practice
- ☐ 10. I actively seek out new experiences
- ☐ 11. When I hear about a new idea or approach I immediately start working out how to apply it in practice

☐ 12. I am keen on self-discipline such as watching my diet, taking regular exercise, sticking to a fixed routine, etc.

☐ 13. I take pride in doing a thorough job

☐ 14. I get on best with logical, analytical people and less well with spontaneous, 'irrational'

☐ 15. I take care over the interpretation of data available to me and avoid jumping to conclusions

☐ 16. I like to reach a decision carefully after weighing up many alternatives

☐ 17. I'm attracted more to novel, unusual ideas than to practical ones

☐ 18. I don't like disorganised things and prefer to fit things into a coherent pattern

☐ 19. I accept and stick to laid down procedures and policies so long as I regard them as an efficient way of getting the job done

☐ 20. I like to relate my actions to a general principle

☐ 21. In discussions I like to get straight to the point

☐ 22. I tend to have distant, rather formal relationships with people at work

☐ 23. I thrive on the challenge of tackling something new and different

☐ 24. I enjoy fun-loving, spontaneous people

☐ 25. I pay meticulous attention to detail before coming to a conclusion

☐ 26. I find it difficult to produce ideas on impulse

☐ 27. I believe in coming to the point immediately

☐ 28. I am careful not to jump to conclusions too quickly

☐ 29. I prefer to have as many resources of information as possible – the more data to think over the better

☐ 30. Flippant people who don't take things seriously enough usually irritate me

☐ 31. I listen to other people's points of view before putting my own forward

☐ 32. I tend to be open about how I'm feeling

☐ 33. In discussions I enjoy watching the manoeuvrings of the other participants

☐ 34. I prefer to respond to events on a spontaneous, flexible basis rather than plan things out in advance

☐ 35. I tend to be attracted to techniques such as network analysis, flow charts, branching programs, contingency planning, etc.

☐ 36. It worries me if I have to rush out a piece of work to meet a tight deadline

☐ 37. I tend to judge people's ideas on their practical merits

☐ 38. Quiet, thoughtful people tend to make me feel uneasy

☐ 39. I often get irritated by people who want to rush things

☐ 40. It is more important to enjoy the present moment than to think about the past or future

☐ 41. I think that decisions based on a thorough analysis of all the information are sounder than those based on intuition

☐ 42. I tend to be a perfectionist

☐ 43. In discussions I usually produce lots of spontaneous ideas

☐ 44. In meetings I put forward practical realistic ideas

☐ 45. More often than not, rules are there to be broken

☐ 46. I prefer to stand back from a situation

☐ 47. I can often see inconsistencies and weaknesses in other people's arguments

☐ 48. On balance I talk more than I listen

☐ 49. I can often see better, more practical ways to get things done

☐ 50. I think written reports should be short and to the point

☐ 51. I believe that rational, logical thinking should win the day

☐ 52. I tend to discuss specific things with people rather than engaging in social discussion

☐ 53. I like people who approach things realistically rather than theoretically

☐ 54. In discussions I get impatient with irrelevancies and digressions

☐ 55. If I have a report to write I tend to produce lots of drafts before settling on the final version

☐ 56. I am keen to try things out to see if they work in practice

☐ 57. I am keen to reach answers via a logical approach

☐ 58. I enjoy being the one that talks a lot

☐ 59. In discussions I often find I am the realist, keeping people to the point and avoiding wild speculations

☐ 60. I like to ponder many alternatives before making up my mind

☐ 61. In discussions with people I often find I am the most dispassionate and objective

☐ 62. In discussions I'm more likely to adopt a 'low profile' than to take the lead and do most of the talking

☐ 63. I like to be able to relate current actions to a longer term bigger picture

☐ 64. When things go wrong I am happy to shrug it off and 'put it down to experience'

☐ 65. I tend to reject wild, spontaneous ideas as being impractical

☐ 66. It's best to think carefully before taking action

☐ 67. On balance I do the listening rather than the talking

☐ 68. I tend to be tough on people who find it difficult to adopt a logical approach

☐ 69. Most times I believe the end justifies the means

☐ 70. I don't mind hurting people's feelings so long as the job gets done

☐ 71. I find the formality of having specific objectives and plans stifling

☐ 72. I'm usually one of the people who puts life into a party

☐ 73. I do whatever is expedient to get the job done

☐ 74. I quickly get bored with methodical, detailed work

☐ 75. I am keen on exploring the basic assumptions, principles and theories underpinning things and events

☐ 76. I'm always interested to find out what people think
☐ 77. I like meetings to be run on methodical lines, sticking to laid down agenda, etc.
☐ 78. I steer clear of subjective or ambiguous topics
☐ 79. I enjoy the drama and excitement of a crisis situation
☐ 80. People often find me insensitive to their feelings

Scoring and interpreting the learning styles questionnaire

The questionnaire is scored by awarding one point for each ticked item. There are no points for crossed items. Simply indicate on the lists below which items were ticked by circling the appropriate question number.

2	7	1	5
4	13	3	9
6	15	8	11
10	16	12	19
17	25	14	21
23	28	18	27
24	29	20	35
32	31	22	37
34	33	26	44
38	36	30	49
40	39	42	50
43	41	47	53
45	46	51	54
48	52	57	56
58	55	61	59
64	60	63	65
71	62	68	69
72	66	75	70
74	67	77	73
79	76	78	80

TOTALS

| Activist | Reflector | Theorist | Pragmatist |

Plot the totals on the arms of the cross below:

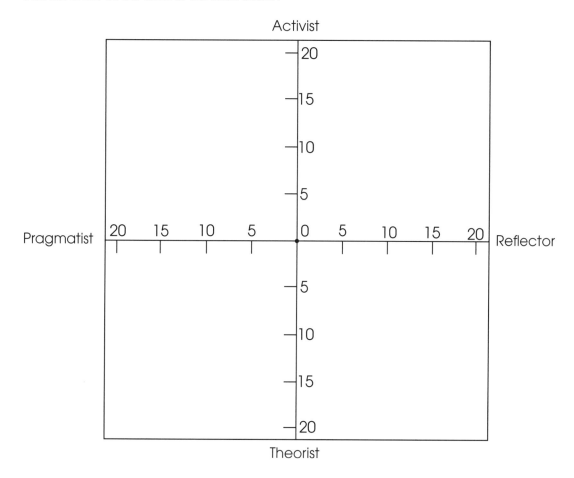

Your result may show that you have a particular learning style preference.

It may be useful to bear this in mind as you approach coaching relationships. How does the approach you adopt impact on your thoughts and actions? How might learning style theory affect your coaching relationships? If you have a coachee with another learning style, how best can you support them to improve their performance?

At this point you may also find it helpful to read through the 'Learning styles – general descriptions' which follow. These descriptions provide more detail and should help you clarify your sense of your own preferred style(s).

Appendix 2

Learning styles – general descriptions

Activists

Activists involve themselves fully and without bias in new experiences. They enjoy the 'here and now' and are happy to be dominated by immediate experiences. They are open-minded, not sceptical, and this tends to make them enthusiastic about anything new. Their philosophy is: 'I'll try anything once'. They tend to act first and consider the consequences later. Their days are filled with activity. They tackle problems by brainstorming. As soon as the excitement from one activity has died down, they are busy looking for the next. They tend to thrive on the challenge of new experiences but are bored by implementation and longer-term consolidation. They are gregarious people, constantly involving themselves with others; but, in doing so, they seek to centre all activities on themselves.

Reflectors

Reflectors like to stand back to ponder experiences and observe them from many different perspectives. They collect data (both first-hand and from others) and prefer to think about it thoroughly before coming to any conclusion. The thorough collection and analysis of data about experiences and events is what counts for them so they tend to postpone reaching definitive conclusions for as long as possible. Their philosophy is to be cautious. They are thoughtful people who like to consider all possible angles and implications before making a move. They prefer to take a back seat in meetings and discussions. They enjoy observing other people in action. They listen to others and get the drift of the discussion before making their own points. They tend to adopt a low profile and have a slightly distant, tolerant unruffled air about them. When they act, it is part of a wide picture, which includes the past as well as the present and others' observations as well as their own.

Theorists

Theorists adapt and integrate observations into complex but logically sound theories. They think problems through, in a vertical, step-by-step, logical way. They assimilate disparate facts into coherent theories. They tend to be perfectionists who won't rest easy until things are tidy and fit into a rational scheme. They like to analyse and synthesise. They are keen on basic assumptions, principles, theories, models and systems. Their philosophy prizes rationality and logic. 'If it's logical it's good'. Questions they frequently ask include: 'Does it make sense?' 'How does this fit with that?' 'What are the basic assumptions?' They tend to be detached, analytical and dedicated to rational objectivity rather than anything subjective or ambiguous. Their approach to problems is consistently logical. This is their 'mind set' and they rigidly reject anything that doesn't fit with it. They prefer to maximise certainty and they feel uncomfortable with subjective judgments, lateral thinking and anything flippant.

Pragmatists

Pragmatists are keen on trying out ideas, theories and techniques to see if they work in practice. They positively search out new ideas and take the first opportunity to experiment with applications. They are the sort of people who return from management courses brimming with new ideas that they want to try out in practice. They like to get on with things and they act quickly and confidently on ideas that attract them. They tend to get impatient with ruminating and open-ended discussions. They are essentially practical, down-to-earth people who like making practical decisions and solving problems. They respond to problems and opportunities 'as a challenge'. Their philosophy is: 'There is always a better way' and 'if it works it's good'.

In descending order of likelihood, the most common combinations are:

1st   Reflector/Theorist

2nd   Theorist/ Pragmatist

3rd   Reflector/Pragmatist

4th   Activist/Pragmatist

Learning styles – a further perspective

Activists

Activists learn best from activities where:

- There are new experiences/problems/opportunities from which to learn
- They can engross themselves in short 'here and now' activities such as business games, competitive teamwork tasks, role-playing exercises
- There is excitement/drama/crisis and things chop and change with a range of diverse activities to tackle
- They have a lot of limelight/high visibility, i.e. they can 'chair' meetings, lead discussions, and give presentations
- They are allowed to generate ideas without being constrained by policy or structure or feasibility
- They are 'thrown in at the deep end' with a task they think is difficult, i.e. when set a challenge with inadequate resources and adverse conditions
- They are involved with other people, i.e. bouncing ideas off them, solving problems as part of a team
- It is appropriate to 'have a go'.

Activists learn least from, and may react against, activities where:

- Learning involves a passive role, i.e. listening to lectures, monologues, explanations, statements of how things should be done, reading, watching
- They are asked to stand back and not be involved
- They are required to assimilate, analyse and interpret lots of 'messy' data
- They are required to engage in solitary work, i.e. reading, writing, thinking on their own
- They are asked to assess beforehand what they will learn, and to appraise afterwards what they have learned
- They are offered statements they see as 'theoretical', i.e. explanations of cause or background
- They are asked to repeat essentially the same activity over and over again, i.e. when practising
- They have precise instructions to follow, with little room for manoeuvre

- They are asked to do a thorough job, i.e. attend to detail, tie up loose ends, 'dot the i's and cross the t's'.

Summary of strengths:

- Flexible and open-minded
- Happy to have a go
- Happy to be exposed to new situations
- Optimistic about anything new and therefore unlikely to resist change.

Summary of weaknesses:

- Tend to take the immediately obvious action without thinking
- Often take unnecessary risks
- Tend to do too much themselves and hog the limelight
- Rush into action without sufficient preparation
- Get bored with implementation/consolidation.

Key questions for activists:

- Shall I learn something new, i.e. that I didn't know/couldn't do before?
- Will there be a wide variety of different activities? (I don't want to sit and listen for more than an hour at a stretch!)
- Will it be OK to have a go/let my hair down/make mistakes/have fun?
- Will I encounter some tough problems and challenges?
- Will there be other like-minded people to mix with?

Reflectors

Reflectors learn best from activities where:

- They are allowed or encouraged to watch/think/chew over activities
- They are able to stand back from events and listen/observe, i.e. observing a group at work, taking a back seat in a meeting, watching a film or video
- They are allowed to think before acting, to assimilate before commencing, i.e. given time to prepare, a chance to read in advance a brief giving background data
- They can carry out some painstaking research, i.e. investigate, assemble information, and probe to get to the bottom of things
- They have the opportunity to review what has happened, and what they have learned
- They are asked to produce carefully considered analyses and reports
- They are helped to exchange views with other people without danger, i.e. by prior agreement, within a structured learning experience
- They can reach a decision in their own time, without pressure and tight deadlines.

Reflectors learn least from, and may react against, activities where:

- They are 'forced' into the limelight, i.e. to act as leader/chairman, to role-play in front of onlookers
- They are involved in situations which require action without planning
- They are pitched into doing something without warning, i.e. to produce an instant reaction, to produce an off-the-top-of-the-head idea
- They are given insufficient data on which to base a conclusion
- They are given cut-and-dried instructions on how things should be done
- They are worried by time pressures or rushed from one activity to another
- In the interests of expediency, they have to make short cuts or do a superficial job.

Summary of strengths:

- Careful
- Thorough and methodical
- Thoughtful
- Good at listening to others and assimilating information
- Rarely jump to conclusions.

Summary of weaknesses:

- Tend to hold back from direct participation
- Slow to make up their minds and reach a decision
- Tend to be too cautious and not take enough risks
- Not assertive – they aren't particularly forthcoming and have no 'small talk'.

Key questions for reflectors:

- Will I be given adequate time to consider, assimilate and prepare?
- Will there be opportunities/facilities to assemble relevant information?
- Will there be opportunities to listen to other people's viewpoints – preferably a wide cross-section of people with a variety of views?
- Will I be under pressure to be slapdash or to extemporise?

Theorists

Theorists learn best from activities where:

- What is being offered is part of a system, model, concept or theory
- They have time to explore methodically the associations and inter-relationships between ideas, events and situations
- They have a chance to question and probe the basic methodology, assumptions or logic behind something, i.e. by taking part in a question and answer session, or by checking a paper for inconsistencies

- They are intellectually stretched, i.e. by analysing a complex situation, being tested in a tutorial session, by teaching high-calibre people who ask searching questions
- They are in structured situations with a clear purpose
- They can listen to or read about ideas and concepts that emphasise rationality or logic and are well argued/elegant/watertight
- They can analyse and then generalise the reasons for success or failure
- They are offered interesting ideas and concepts even though they are not immediately relevant
- They are required to understand and participate in complex situations.

Theorists learn least from, and may react against, activities where:
- They are pitched into doing something without a context or apparent purpose
- They have to participate in situations emphasising emotions and feelings
- They are involved in unstructured activities where ambiguity and uncertainty are high, i.e. with open-ended problems, on sensitivity training
- They are asked to act or decide without any basis in policy, principle or concept
- They are faced with a hotchpotch of alternative/contradictory techniques/methods without exploring any in depth, i.e. as on a 'once over lightly' course
- They find the subject matter platitudinous, shallow or gimmicky
- They feel out of tune with other participants, i.e. when they are with lots of activists or people of lower intellectual calibre.

Summary of strengths:
- Logical 'vertical' thinkers
- Rational and objective
- Good at asking probing questions
- Disciplined approach.

Summary of weaknesses:
- Restricted in lateral thinking
- Low tolerance for uncertainty, disorder and ambiguity
- Intolerant of anything subjective or intuitive
- Full of 'shoulds', 'oughts' and 'musts'.

Key questions for theorists:
- Will there be lots of opportunities to ask questions?
- Do the objectives and the programme of events indicate a clear structure and purpose?
- Will I encounter complex ideas and concepts that are likely to stretch me?
- Are the approaches to be used and concepts to be explored 'respectable', i.e. sound and valid?
- Will I be with people of similar intellectual calibre to myself?

Pragmatists

Pragmatists learn best from activities where:

- There is an obvious link between the subject matter and a problem or opportunity at work
- They are shown techniques for doing things with obvious practical advantages, i.e. how to save time, how to make a good first impression, how to deal with awkward people
- They have a chance to try out and practise techniques with coaching/feedback from a credible expert, i.e. someone who is successful and can do the techniques themselves
- They are exposed to a model they can emulate, i.e. a respected boss, a demonstration from someone with a proven track record, lots of examples/anecdotes, and a film showing how it's done
- They are given techniques currently applicable to their own job
- They are given immediate opportunities to implement what they have learned
- There is a high face validity in the learning activity, i.e. a good simulation, 'real' problems
- They can concentrate on practical issues, i.e. drawing up action plans with an obvious end product, suggesting short cuts, giving tips.

Pragmatists learn least from, and may react against, activities where:

- The learning is not related to an immediate need they recognise/they cannot see, an immediate relevance/practical benefit
- Organisers of the learning, or the event itself, seems distant from reality, i.e. 'ivory towered', all theory and general principles, pure 'chalk and talk'
- There is no practice or clear guidelines on how to do it
- They feel that people are 'going round in circles' and not getting anywhere fast enough
- There are political, managerial or personal obstacles to implementation
- There is no apparent reward from the learning activity, i.e. more sales, shorter meetings, higher bonus, promotion.

Summary of strengths:

- Keen to test things out in practice
- Practical, down to earth, realistic
- Businesslike – gets straight to the point
- Technique oriented.

Summary of weaknesses:

- Tend to reject anything without an obvious application
- Not very interested in theory or basic principles
- Tend to seize on the first expedient solution to a problem
- Impatient with waffle
- On balance, task oriented not people oriented.

Key questions for pragmatists:

- Will there be ample opportunities to practise and experiment?
- Will there be lots of practical tips and techniques?
- Will we be addressing real problems and will this result in action plans to tackle some of my current problems?
- Will we be exposed to experts who know how to/can do it themselves?

Index